D1742486

MCQ TUTOR
for
PRIMARY FRCS

MCQ TUTOR
for
PRIMARY FRCS

Basic Science for Surgeons

Michael Hobsley, TD, PhD, MChir, FRCS
Professor of Surgical Science, The Middlesex Hospital Medical School and Consultant Surgeon, The Middlesex Hospital, London; lately Examiner in Applied Physiology for the Primary FRCS Examination and Penrose May Tutor of the Royal College of Surgeons of England.

Peter Abrahams, MB, BS
Lecturer in Anatomy, The Middlesex Hospital Medical School, London.

Brian Cardell, MD, FRCPath.
Reader in Morbid Anatomy, King's College Hospital Medical School, London; lately Examiner in Pathology for the Primary FRCS Examination of the Royal College of Surgeons of England.

WILLIAM HEINEMANN MEDICAL BOOKS LTD
London

First published 1980

©Michael Hobsley, Peter Abrahams, and Brian Cardell, 1980

ISBN 0 433 15005

Filmset by Reproduction Drawings Ltd., Sutton, Surrey
Printed in Great Britain by McCorquodale (Newton) Ltd.,
Merseyside

CONTENTS

Contents

PREFACE

The Royal Colleges of Surgeons of the British Isles and of Australasia all require candidates for their Fellowship to pass a Primary examination in the basic sciences of anatomy, physiology and pathology before proceeding to the final examination. All these Colleges include, as part of this Primary or Part I examination, a paper of Multiple Choice Questions. In the two Scottish Colleges, this MCQ element constitutes one of only two modes of testing, the other being an oral examination. In the English and Irish Colleges, there is also a written paper. The Australasian College has, apart from its MCQ paper, only an interview. Thus to varying degrees it is nevertheless true for all these Colleges that the MCQ paper is of great importance.

This book is a collection of about eighty questions in each of the three disciplines. The format of the questions remains the same throughout: they consist of a stem followed by five completions. The stem is to be read in turn with each of the completions, and the candidate has to decide whether the complete statement resulting from the combination of the stem with that completion is true or false. It is important to realise that each completion may result in a true or a false statement, so that all five statements may be true or all five may be false, or any intermediate number between zero and five may be true, the rest false. This system is in sharp contrast to the one in which the answer that is *most* correct, and not necessarily the *only* one that is correct, is to be marked.

This particular format is the one used by the English College, and so to an extent the book is aimed at those who propose to take the Primary of the English College. The differences in format between the English and the other Colleges are relatively minor, and with the proviso that the candidate must naturally familiarize himself with the style of the paper set in the College of his choice, he will find the questions in this book valuable and useful for practice.

There is no doubt that this element of practice is important, as anyone will testify who can remember his first experience of trying to cope with a MCQ type of paper. However, in all three disciplines the authors of these questions are trying to do more than provide practice in answering the questions. One further aim is to provide the student with a check on the progress he is making in acquiring the necessary knowledge. Another aim is to teach: to probe deeply for gaps in knowledge and to fill those gaps with information, often of a type that is not readily found in text-books. This aspect is particularly important in physiology, because at least in the British Isles there is no single

Preface

text that is generally accepted as the best in the field. Remember that the subject being examined is not physiology, but physiology *applied to surgery*. By contrast, there are accepted texts for applied anatomy and pathology. It is for this reason that the notes given with the answer key tend to be longer in physiology than in the two other disciplines.

Learning anatomy certainly strains the power of memory; indeed the student often complains that he cannot see the point of learning the minutiae of topographical anatomy in the way his teachers seem to accept. Yet the topographical foundation is often all-important to understanding the clinical problem. For this reason, in the section on anatomy Dr. Abrahams has sometimes prefaced the stem with a brief explanation of the clinical application of the relevant subject.

Every student will find his own way of using this book to his best possible advantage. He may, however, find the following suggestions of some help. The questions are always separated from the correct answer key and the commentaries by the necessity of having to turn a page (occasionally more than one): this arrangement will facilitate self-marking of his answers. On a separate sheet of paper he should write down T for True if he thinks a completion is correct, F for False if he thinks the statement is incorrect, or leave a blank if he cannot make up his mind whether the completion is true or false. In due course he can look up the answer key and award himself one mark for every answer he makes that agrees with the key (whether that answer be True or False), he deducts a mark for every answer which is in disagreement with the key, and the 'don't know' answers score nothing, either positive or negative. Thus the top mark possible for a question of five completions is 5.

In very approximate terms, a candidate may consider his performance reasonably satisfactory if he can achieve a score of over 50 per cent, i.e. 25 marks out of 50 for a section of ten questions. If he then studies the commentaries, make sure that the answers he got right were selected by him for the right reasons, and that he understands the reasons for his incorrect choice in the case of the answers he got wrong, then he is getting the maximum gain from the book. Moreover, a repetition of the self-examination on that section in two weeks' time should result in a better score, thus enabling the student to quantify his progress. The proof that his knowledge and preparedness for the real examination are improving can be a real encouragement.

The Editor's contribution of questions on applied physiology have been criticised by several experts in their various fields, and the contributions in anatomy and pathology have also been independently scrutinised. Thus the authors hope that the answers to the questions will prove to be reliable and acceptable to experts. Differences in interpretation of the wording of the stem and completions are always possible, and comments and criticisms are welcome.

It remains only to express the best wishes of the authors to the reader for success in his studies.

I. ANATOMY

1. HEAD AND NECK

A dental surgeon is unlucky during the removal of a lower wisdom tooth and bruises the lingual nerve. At your clinic the patient's complaints may include:-

A. loss of sensation in the lower jaw teeth
B. lack of sensation in the gums of his lower jaw
C. an area of numbness over the chin and lower lip
D. a slightly dry mouth
E. a diminished sense of taste in the posterior portion of the tongue.

Answers overleaf

A. FALSE   Lower jaw teeth sensation is supplied by the inferior alveolar nerve, which like the lingual, is a branch of the mandibular nerve and often runs parallel to it prior to entering the bone at the mandibular foramen.

B. TRUE   The lingual nerve is sensory to the anterior two thirds of the tongue, i.e. that portion anterior to the sulcus terminalis, as well as to the floor of the mouth and the gums of the lower jaw.

C. FALSE   Numbness in the skin of the chin is due to a lesion of the mental nerve. This nerve is a sensory terminal branch of the inferior alveolar nerve. It leaves the jaw by the mental foramen which is easily found on the skeleton just inferior to the canine/pre-molar teeth. It is this area of numbness that is felt following an inferior alveolar (dental) block and makes one think the lip has grown to twice its size!

D. & E.   TRUE and FALSE   A reduced secretion from the sub-mandibular and sublingual glands on one side will not always be noticeable. However, if tested with lemon drops, it can be shown that following a lingual nerve lesion medial to the 3rd molar tooth there is indeed a reduced or absent secretion. This is readily explained by the fact that the chorda tympani joins the lingual nerve proximally in the infratemporal fossa and is consequently also damaged in this lesion. The chorda tympani carries preganglionic parasympathetic secreto-motor fibres to the submandibular ganglion. It also contains taste fibres from the anterior two thirds of the tongue whose cells of origin are within the petrous temporal bone. The taste fibres to the posterior part of the tongue are carried by the glossopharyngeal nerve (IX). Those taste buds around the valleculae and epiglottis are supplied by the vagus (X).

Parasympathetic post-ganglionic fibres are carried by the:-

A. auriculotemporal nerve
B. long ciliary nerves
C. greater superficial petrosal nerve
D. chorda tympani
E. deep petrosal nerve.

Answers overleaf

H & N2 Answers

A. TRUE   Parasympathetic nerve fibres are contained in cranial nerves III, VII, IX and X and sacral nerves 2,3, and 4. The pre-ganglionic fibres are carried by the tympanic branch of IX via the tympanic plexus and lesser superficial petrosal nerve, through the foramen ovale to the otic ganglion. Following synapse within the ganglion the post-ganglionic fibres are then carried by the auriculotemporal nerve to the parotid gland where they are secretomotor.

B. FALSE   The long ciliary nerves are mixed sensory and sympathetic, being a continuation of the nasociliary nerve. They accompany the dozen or more short ciliary nerves which are carrying the parasympathetic post-ganglionic fibres from the ciliary ganglion to the ciliary muscle and sphincter pupillae.

C. & D FALSE   The greater superficial petrosal nerve carries pre-ganglionic parasympathetic fibres from the nervus intermedius of the facial nerve to the pterygopalatine ganglion where they synapse. The post-ganglionic fibres leave the ganglion via the zygomatic and palatine nerves to the lacrimal and palatine glands respectively. The pterygopalatine ganglion is the ganglion of 'hay fever' causing the eyes to water and the nose to run, and the palate to secrete mucus. The chorda tympani also carries pre-ganglionic fibres of VII but these are destined for the submandibular ganglion and hence to the submandibular and sublingual glands.

E. FALSE   The deep petrosal nerve is carrying mainly sympathetic fibres which have come via the superior cervical ganglion, and the internal carotid artery plexus. Within the carotid canal the deep petrosal nerve branches off to join with the greater superficial petrosal (See C) thereby forming the nerve of the pterygoid canal. This nerve with both parasympathetic and sympathetic fibres runs into the pterygoid canal.

A patient has an invasive tumour within the cavernous sinus. It is causing pressure on the nerves that leave the sinus and pass through the superior orbital fissure. Presenting signs in this patient may include:-

A. a much dilated pupil
B. a drooped eyelid (ptosis)
C. an eye which cannot abduct from the resting position
D. a weakness in screwing up the eyes tightly
E. an eye which is directed to look downwards and laterally.

It is always taught that the scalp has five layers and a rich anastomosis of vessels and nerves. Nerves and arteries in the scalp include:-

A. small twigs from the infraorbital nerve
B. the posterior auricular artery
C. the greater auricular nerve
D. the posterior primary ramus of C1
E. the supratrochlear artery.

Answers overleaf

H & N3 Answers

A. & B TRUE The nerves which are found in the sinus are cranial nerves III, IV, VI and the ophthalmic division of V. There are also some sympathetic fibres around the carotid artery. A lesion of the third cranial nerve would paralyse all the ocular muscles except superior oblique and lateral rectus. It would also cause ptosis due to the striated muscle portion of levator palpebrae (See TH 9) and paralyse the ciliary muscle and sphincter pupillae. These last two muscles are in fact parasympathetic-innervated, the post-ganglionic fibres from the ciliary ganglion being carried by the III nerve division to the inferior oblique muscle.

C. This is typical of a VI nerve lesion (abducent nerve) and is due to paralysis of the lateral rectus muscle.

D. FALSE The ability to shut the eyes tightly is a function of orbicularis oculi which is innervated by the VII (facial) nerve. This nerve does not enter either the cavernous sinus or the superior orbital fissure. It leaves the skull via the petrous temporal bone and the stylomastoid foramen.

E. TRUE (See A above). This is seen in a IIIrd nerve lesion as the only muscles intact are superior oblique (IV) and lateral rectus (VI) which together pull the eye down and outwards.

H & N4 Answers

A. FALSE The infraorbital nerve is a branch of the maxillary division of the trigeminal and it is the zygomatico-temporal branch that helps supply the scalp. In fact each division of the trigeminal nerve is represented—supraorbital and supratrochlear (Vi) and auriculotemporal (Viii).

B. TRUE This is one of the three branches of the external carotid that supply the scalp. The other arteries involved are the superficial temporal and occipital.

C. FALSE This nerve which originates from C2, 3 supplies the ear, as well as the mastoid, parotid and masseter regions. It does not reach the scalp.

D. FALSE C1 does not normally have a cutaneous branch

E. TRUE The supratrochlear and supraorbital arteries are both branches of the internal carotid artery via its ophthalmic branch. These anastomose with the external carotid branches (See B).

The posterior triangle of the neck:-

A. has for its floor levator scapulae, splenius and scalene muscles
B. contains posterior rami of C 2 3 and 4
C. is covered by the deep cervical investing fascia embedded in which lies the accessory nerve
D. contains a large group of lymph nodes lying along the accessory nerve
E. is bounded posteriorly by the posterior border of trapezius muscle.

Answers overleaf

H & N5 Answers

A. TRUE The muscles of the floor consist from above downwards of semispinalis capitis, splenius, levator scapulae, scaleni posterior and medius and if the sternomastoid is pulled forward, scalenus anterior. This muscular floor is covered by a fascial carpet. The carpet is a part of the prevertebral fascia of the neck and also contributes to the formation of the axillary sheath as the subclavian vessels pick up the fascia on leaving the triangle. This fascial carpet also acts as protection to the nerves to the rhomboids, levator scapulae, the long thoracic nerve, and the phrenic nerve. If the carpet is intact these nerves are undamaged.

B. FALSE You should know this trick by now! (H&N 4D Answer). The cutaneous nerves of the posterior triangle are anterior primary rami of C2, 3, 4. The posterior rami are concerned with the back muscles, suboccipital triangle muscles and the greater occipital nerve (C2) which is sensory. The anterior primary rami of C 2 3 4 radiate from the posterior border of sternomastoid as the lesser occipital (C 2,3) and supraclavicular (C 3,4).

C. TRUE This polo-neck, collar-like investing fascia covers the posterior triangle, splits around trapezius and sternomastoid, and attaches to the clavicle.

D. TRUE Lying in the fat between the investing fascial roof and fascial carpet lie the lateral group of inferior deep cervical or supraclavicular nodes. These drain the scalp and neck and because of their close relationship to the accessory nerve the latter may be involved in lymph node pathology.

E. FALSE The posterior border of the posterior triangle is the anterior border of the trapezius.

You are presented with a patient whose problem is that of crying, not of emotional but of anatomical origin. You decide to examine the pathway of tears from production to disposal. In formulating your differential diagnosis you remember that the:-

A. lacrimal gland lies in a shallow groove in the lacrimal bone
B. parasympathetic secretomotor fibres to the lacrimal gland are carried via the greater petrosal nerve and relay in the sphenopalatine ganglion
C. arterial supply to the gland is from a branch of the external carotid artery
D. nasolacrimal duct lies in a bony canal formed by the maxilla, lacrimal bone and inferior concha
E. nasolacrimal duct opens into the hiatus semilunaris in the lateral wall of the nose.

H & N7 Questions

The surgeon performing thyroidectomy should remember that the:-

A. recurrent laryngeal nerve is an intimate relation of the inferior thyroid artery
B. recurrent laryngeal nerve supplies all the intrinsic muscles of the larynx
C. superior laryngeal nerve supplies the cricothyroid muscle
D. inferior thyroid artery is a branch of the costocervical trunk of the subclavian
E. inferior thyroid artery is quite short and very straight.

Answers overleaf

H & N6 Answers

A. FALSE   The gland lies in the zygomatic process of the frontal bone and consists of two parts hooked around the free edge of levator palpebrae superioris.

B. TRUE   These fibres are from the seventh cranial nerve (See H & N2).

C. FALSE   The lacrimal artery is a lateral branch of the ophthalmic artery which is itself a branch of the internal carotid artery.

D. & E.   TRUE and FALSE   The nasolacrimal duct opens into the lateral wall of the nose under the inferior concha. The hiatus semilunaris is a curved groove in the middle meatus related to the openings of the frontal and maxillary sinuses.

H & N7 Answers

A. TRUE   Near the lower pole of the thyroid gland the recurrent laryngeal nerve is always in close contact with the inferior thyroid artery. Numerous dissections reveal that the exact relationship is variable; sometimes the nerve even winds through branches of the artery

B. & C   FALSE and TRUE   The recurrent laryngeal nerve supplies all intrinsic muscles except the cricothyroid which is supplied by the external laryngeal branch of the superior laryngeal nerve.

D. FALSE   The inferior thyroid artery is a branch of the thyrocervical trunk which comes off the first part of the subclavian artery.

E. FALSE   It is quite long and always tortuous, often having a 'C' shaped loop. As the thyroid is encased in the pretracheal fascia it rises on swallowing and therefore pulls up the artery which must be able to cope with this necessary increased length. If it were straight and short one might rupture it on swallowing.

With regard to the paranasal sinuses:-

A. in the newborn the maxillary sinus is relatively large compared to the adult
B. the mucous membrane of the maxillary sinus and the upper premolar teeth have the same nerve supply
C. referred pain from the frontal sinus may be experienced as far back as the vertex
D. the sphenoidal sinuses are supplied by the posterior ethmoidal nerves
E. the frontal, sphenoidal, maxillary and anterior ethmoidal sinuses all drain into the middle meatus.

A neurologist informs you that his patient has a tumour in the middle ear, situated along the posterior wall. On examining the patient yourself, you decide that he is possibly correct as you find that:-

A. the patient has abnormal taste sensation in the anterior ⅔ of his tongue and reduced secretions in the mouth
B. stapedius muscle seems damaged
C. he is drooling from the corner of the mouth
D. his auditory tube seems blocked
E. his internal carotid arterial flow is restricted at this level.

Answers overleaf

H & N8 Answers

A. FALSE   The paranasal air sinuses are only rudimentary in the newborn. Of particular clinical importance is the fact that the mastoid air cells, because of their lack of development, cannot protect the facial nerve as it leaves the stylomastoid foramen. This explains why facial palsy is not rare following forceps delivery

B. TRUE   The superior alveolar (dental) nerve supplies both structures and it is quite common for a dentist to perform some procedure, such as filling, when the true cause of the pain is within the sinus. (See H & N1).

C. TRUE   The nerve supply is by the supraorbital nerve which carries up onto the scalp as far as the vertex. Referred pain to the scalp may be a presenting feature of frontal sinusitis.

D. TRUE

E. FALSE   All except the sphenoidal sinus do indeed drain into the middle meatus. The sphenoidal sinus drains into the sphenoethmoidal recess.

H & N9 Answers

A. B. & C. TRUE   It is evident from these questions that he has damage of the facial nerve—causing buccinator paralysis (drooling); damage to the nerve to stapedius which causes hyperacusis; and damage to his chorda tympani nerve causing taste and salivary problems. The facial nerve and these branches all lie within the petrous temporal bone immediately posterior to the posterior wall of the middle ear.

D. FALSE   For his auditory tube to be blocked the anterior wall would be involved. The opening in the posterior wall is the aditus to the mastoid antrum and mastoid air cells.

E. FALSE   The internal carotid artery and its sympathetic plexus lie at the anterior inferior corner of the middle ear. Close to the posterior wall lies the sigmoid sinus and clinically one must remember this relationship when dealing with possible spread of infection from a mastoiditis.

Fascial planes of the neck are of considerable surgical importance with regard to both operative dissections and the spread of infection. Features of the fasciae of the neck include that the:-

A. superficial fascia contains platysma, external and anterior jugular veins
B. pretracheal fascia extends as far inferiorly as the fibrous pericardium
C. prevertebral fascia extends from the base of the skull into the axilla
D. deep cervical, investing fascia lies only deep to the parotid gland
E. sympathetic chain lies between the carotid sheath and the deep cervical, investing fascia.

Answers overleaf

H & N10 Answers

A. TRUE   The superficial fascia is only a thin layer on the neck containing the veins, decussating fibres of platysma, and in some individuals a considerable amount of adipose tissue.

B. TRUE   The pretracheal fascia extends from the cricoid and thyroid cartilages above to the pericardium below. It binds the thyroid gland to the larynx.

C. TRUE   The prevertebral fascia lies posterior to the oesophagus covering the vertebrae and prevertebral muscles from the base of skull down to the posterior mediastinum where it blends with the anterior longitudinal ligament of the upper thorax. Laterally this fascia covers the scalene muscles, and where the brachial plexus and subclavian artery leave the neck the axillary sheath is formed.

D. FALSE   The deep cervical, investing fascia lies like a polo-neck collar from the mandible, zygomatic arch, mastoid process and superior nuchal line above, to the manubrium, clavicle, acromion and scapular spine below. It splits around trapezius, sternomastoid, the strap muscles and parotid glands. The fact that it encases the parotid gland helps explain the pain of an enlarged gland such as during a mumps infection.

E. FALSE   The sympathetic chain lies just posterior to the carotid sheath but just anterior to the prevertebral fascia. During dissection it is often found embedded within the prevertebral fascia.

2. UPPER LIMB

Your patient has sustained a dislocation of the shoulder and a fracture of the greater tubercle of the humerus. The muscles primarily affected by this fracture include:-

A. teres major
B. infraspinatus
C. subscapularis
D. supraspinatus
E. teres minor.

Answers overleaf

17

UL1 Answers

A. FALSE   Teres major is a large thick rectangular muscle which originates from a large impression on the dorsum of the inferior angle of the scapula. It inserts not into the greater tubercle but into the crest of the lesser tubercle of the humerus.

B. & D. TRUE   The infraspinatus and supraspinatus muscles arise by fleshy fibres from their respective fossae on the dorsum of the scapula. They are both inserted by tendons into the greater tubercle. These tendons often fuse with the fibrous capsule of the shoulder joint.

C. FALSE   Subscapularis, although one of the rotator cuff muscles, has a multipennate origin in the subscapular fossa. It is inserted into the lesser tubercle, its tendon grooving the anterior border of the glenoid cavity.

E. TRUE   Teres minor muscle is also one of the four rotator cuff muscles, and is quite a small muscle. During dissection it is often difficult to distinguish from infraspinatus, its origin and insertion being very similar to the much larger infraspinatus. It originates from the lateral border of the scapula and inserts by a tendon into the lowest facet on the greater tubercle of the humerus.

After a forearm fracture your patient is unable to flex the terminal phalanx of her thumb, and the terminal phalanges of her index and middle fingers only. You diagnose an injury to the:-

A. median nerve ✓

B. deep branch of the ulnar nerve ✗

C. posterior interosseous nerve ✗

D. superficial radial nerve ✗

E. anterior interosseous nerve. ✓

Answers overleaf

UL2 Answers

A. FALSE   Although at first sight it seems reasonable to think that this is a median nerve problem, it should be obvious that loss of flexion of only the terminal phalanx points to a more specific lesion in the forearm (see E).

B. FALSE   The deep branch of the ulnar nerve originates between the pisiform and hamate and supplies the hypothenar eminence and all the intrinsic muscles of the hand, except the five usually supplied by the median nerve.

C. FALSE   The posterior interosseous nerve, sometimes called the deep radial nerve, originates anterior to the capsule of the elbow and then pierces supinator muscle before proceeding into the posterior compartment to supply extensors of the wrist and fingers

D. FALSE   The superficial radial nerve is the sensory continuation of the radial nerve distal to the origin of the posterior interosseous nerve. It can usually be found deep to brachio-radialis and becomes cutaneous a few centimetres proximal to the styloid process of the radius.

E. TRUE   Flexion of terminal phalanges is by flexor digitorum profundus, the medial two digits being supplied by the ulnar nerve, and the index and middle fingers by the anterior interosseous nerve. This nerve arises from the median nerve a couple of centimetres distal to the elbow and accompanying the anterior interosseous artery, supplies flexor pollicis longus, pronator quadratus and the lateral two digits of flexor digitorum profundus.

20

Following an accident a young carpenter complains of difficulties with rotatory movements of his forearm with a flexed elbow. He informs you that he has no problem tightening screws but great difficulty unscrewing them. This can be explained by damage to the:-

A. median nerve at the wrist
B. radial nerve in the spiral groove of the humerus
C. radial nerve as it pierces the supinator
D. musculocutaneous nerve in the axilla
E. median nerve at the elbow.

Answers overleaf

UL3 Answers

A. B. C. & D. FALSE   It is obvious that this man's problem is associated with pronation—supination movements of the forearm. The anatomical position, with the palms forwards is the supine position and bringing the palm into that position is supination. Pronation is twisting the palm from the palm forwards to palm backwards position. Screwing home a screw with a normal right hand thread is the strong movement of supination. This is carried out mainly by biceps and supinator. The weaker action of pronation is a function of pronator teres and pronator quadratus. Brachioradialis and the lateral long extensors bring the pronated hand to the midprone position of rest—an important action for beer drinking medics!

A. The median nerve in the hand supplies two lumbrical, three small thenar muscles, and some skin below the wrist.

B. & C. The radial nerve supplies all the extensor muscles of the arm and forearm including brachioradialis and supinator, dividing into a cutaneous superficial branch and the deep radial nerve which is motor to wrist and finger extensors.

D. The musculocutaneous nerve arises in the axilla from the lateral cord of the brachial plexus. It supplies coracobrachialis, brachialis and both heads of biceps. Biceps tendon inserts posteriorly into the radial tuberosity and is the strongest supinator as well as acting with brachialis as an elbow flexor.

E. TRUE   This man's problem can be explained by a median nerve injury at the elbow causing paralysis of both pronator muscles. The median nerve leaves the cubital fossa by passing between the two heads of pronator teres, which it supplies, and then lies on the deep aspect of flexor digitorum superficialis until it approaches the wrist. In the cubital fossa it has numerous muscular branches but of particular importance is the anterior interosseous nerve which arises posteriorly. This accompanies the anterior interosseus artery on the front of the membrane and supplies flexor pollicis longus, flexor digitorum profundus and pronator quadratus before ending in the wrist and intercarpal joints.

A glass cutter slips and damages the upper trunk of the brachial plexus. This injury may cause:-

A. a supinated forearm ✓
B. a shoulder which cannot abduct ﹀
C. an extended elbow ﹁
D. reduced power in serratus anterior muscle ✗
E. wasting of the intrinsic hand muscles. ✗

You are asked to locate some anatomical structures in the normal subject. You show your knowledge by demonstrating that the:-

A. bicipital aponeurosis covers the pronator teres muscle ✓
B. subclavian artery is palpable a finger's breadth medial to the tip of the coracoid process ✗
C. brachioradialis muscle contracts when flexing the semi-pronated forearm against resistance with the fist tight closed ✓
D. first dorsal interosseous muscle contracts when the index finger is adducted ✗
E. ulnar artery enters the hand just lateral to pisiform and superficial to the flexor retinaculum. ✓

Answers overleaf

UL4 Answers

A. FALSE   It will cause the arm to be pronated as the upper trunk comprises fibres of C5 and C6 anterior rami and these supply both biceps and supinator which are the major muscles involved in supination. C5, 6, (7) also supply the brachioradialis via the radial nerve which assists in bringing the arm from a pronated position to a mid-prone position, a working position.

B. TRUE   Abduction would be greatly affected as the deltoid supplied by the axillary nerve C5, 6, would be affected. Also, depending upon the exact site of the injury, the suprascapular nerve may be affected, thus weakening supraspinatus, the other muscle involved in abduction.

C. TRUE   The elbow would be extended as the major flexors biceps and brachialis are supplied by the musclocutaneous nerve C5, 6. Rarely, a small lateral portion of brachialis is supplied by the radial nerve C7.

D. FALSE   Although the long thoracic nerve of Bell to serratus anterior has root contributions from C5, 6 and 7, it does not form distal to this lesion but comes directly from the roots of the brachial plexus.

E. FALSE   The intrinsic muscles of the hand are supplied by T1.

UL5 Answers

A. TRUE   The tendon of biceps brachii inserts into the posterior part of the radial tuberosity and hence this muscle is a most important supinator. Its bicipital aponeurosis (grace à dieu fascia) passes medially and spreads out over the pronator teres muscle. It is an important landmark of the cubital fossa offering protection to the median nerve and brachial artery for the over-enthusiastic performer of venepuncture!

B. FALSE   A rather dirty trick to play. Yes, there is a palpable pulse just medial to the coracoid process but it is that of the axillary artery which begins at the lateral border of the first rib.

C. TRUE   Look at a tennis player's arm.

D. FALSE   The first dorsal interosseous muscle is the bulk of the web between thumb and index finger. Dorsal interossei are used for abduction, not adduction. (Palmar AD, Dorsal AB).

E. TRUE   Careful palpation of a thin warm hand will demonstrate this. The pisiform is the inferior protuberance of the hypothenar eminence.

A young boy falls out of a tree onto the pavement below, sustaining a supracondylar fracture of the elbow. On examination there is no dislocation of the elbow joint but an anterior displacement of the proximal humerus. Likely resultant problems include:-

A. weakened abduction of the wrist
B. weakness of opposition of the thumb
C. ischaemia of the forearm flexors
D. an early claw deformity of the little finger
E. a wrist drop.

The arteries of the upper limb are so arranged that:-

A. the common palmar digital arteries arise from the deep palmar arch
B. to stop bleeding in the hand pressure on the radial artery alone will rarely suffice
C. the brachial artery begins at the lower border of teres minor
D. the profunda brachii artery accompanies the axillary nerve
E. the interosseous arteries of the forearm branch off the radial artery, usually below the elbow joint.

Answers overleaf

UL6 Answers

A. & B. TRUE Abduction of the wrist is a synergistic combined action of the flexor and extensor carpi radialis with slight assistance of the long muscles of the thumb from the extensor surface. A supracondylar fracture of this sort may well damage the median nerve and therefore cause problems for the flexor carpi radialis. The median nerve also supplies the thenar muscles including the opponens pollicis.

C. TRUE The displaced fragment of the humerus often causes damage to the brachial artery with obstruction, which leads to ischaemic necrosis of both forearm groups of muscles. As they are bigger the flexors are the muscles mainly affected, resulting in a flexed wrist with extended fingers; however if the wrist is passively extended the fingers tend to flex. This condition of the forearm muscles is called Volkmann's ischaemic contracture.

D. FALSE The ulnar nerve normally lies posterior to the medial epicondyle and is therefore not affected by this fracture.

E. TRUE It is possible, though not often seen clinically, for the fracture fragments to injure the radial nerve as it emerges from between brachioradialis and brachialis in the cubital fossa.

UL7 Answers

A. & B. FALSE and TRUE The common palmar digital arteries arise from the superficial arch which is formed mainly by the ulnar artery, having entered the hand superficial to the flexor retinaculum. There is also a contribution to this arch from the radial artery in about ⅔ of normal subjects. Wounds of the hand involving the arch often require not only pressure or ligature of radial and ulnar arteries, but due to the rich carpal anastomoses even the brachial artery may need to be tied.

C. & D. FALSE The brachial artery begins at the lower border of teres major and continues down the forearm deep to the bicipital aponeurosis until it gives off its radial and ulnar branches in the cubital fossa, below the elbow joint. In the upper arm its major branch is the profunda brachii which accompanies the radial nerve in the spiral groove of the humerus.

E. FALSE The interosseous arteries do commence below the elbow joint but nearly always from the ulnar artery.

On palpation of the wrist one would find that:-

A. the palmaris longus tendon is present in a minority of people only ✓

B. the median nerve can sometimes be rolled over the tendons of flexor digitorum superficialis ✗

C. the superficial radial nerve can often be rolled over the flexor pollicis longus ✗

D. the radial pulse is usually just medial to the tendon of flexor carpi radialis ✗

E. the scaphoid bone lies in the floor of the anatomical snuff box. ✓

UL9 Questions

Correct pairings of a nerve with a lesion produced by damage of that nerve include:-

A. long thoracic nerve — 'Winged scapulae'. ✗

B. C7 — Absent biceps jerk ✗

C. T1 — Motor loss to intrinsic muscles of the hand ✓

D. Ulnar nerve — Pain in the index finger ✗

E. Radial nerve — Supinator jerk absent. ✗

Answers overleaf

UL8 Answers

A. & B. FALSE and TRUE Palmaris longus is present in a majority (80 – 90%) of people though sometimes occurring in only one arm. This atavistic muscle which originates with the other forearm flexors inserts into the palmar fascia. One contribution to humanity is that it usually protects the median nerve lying on its deep aspect. In individuals not possessing this muscle it is often easy to palpate the median nerve and roll it over the flexor digitorum tendons.

C. FALSE The radial nerve can indeed be palpated, but over the extensor pollicis longus as it crosses the roof of the anatomical snuff box.

D. FALSE It is lateral.

E. TRUE It is here that classically pain is felt on palpation of a fractured scaphoid even if the x-rays are initially negative.

UL9 Answers

A. TRUE The long thoracic nerve (Bell) whose roots are C5 (mainly), C6 and C7 supplies one muscle—serratus anterior. This muscle holds the scapula flat against the back, by inserting into the medial edge of the scapula, and it stabilizes the shoulder joint during abduction. Lesions of this nerve result in the patients complaining of difficulty in combing hair and pulling on clothes and the scapula can be seen to protrude.

B. FALSE Lesions of C7 cause an absence of the triceps reflex arc, not the biceps jerk which is innervated by C5.

C. TRUE All small muscles of the hand are innervated by T1 though in some people C8 innervates the thenar muscles.

D. FALSE An ulnar nerve lesion would cause pain in the region of the little finger and palm of the hand distal to the wrist. Median nerve lesions cause pain in the index finger.

E. TRUE A radial nerve lesion such as caused by a crutch or fractured humeral shaft would cause an absence of both triceps and supinator jerks.

Due to the extreme mobility of the shoulder joint temporary occlusion of the axillary artery may occur. It is also a frequent site of arterial laceration. It is therefore most appropriate that there are arterial anastomoses around the scapula which include the:-

A. subscapular branch of the subclavian artery   ✗
B. suprascapular branch of the thyrocervical trunk, which arises from the first part of the subclavian artery   ✗
C. deep branch of the superficial cervical artery   ✗
D. acromial branch of the thoraco-acromial artery   ✗
E. dorsal scapular artery which often arises from the third part of the subclavian artery.   ✗

Answers overleaf

UL10 Answers

A. B. & C. FALSE, TRUE and TRUE   The subscapular and its major branch the circumflex scapular artery are indeed involved in the scapular anastomosis but arise from the axillary artery, third part. In fact the subscapular artery is the largest branch of the axillary and often anastomoses with the suprascapular artery and superficial cervical artery, both of which originate from the thyrocervical trunk of the subclavian.

D. TRUE   The thoraco-acromial artery arises from the second part of the axillary artery and gives off its pectoral, deltoid, clavicular and acromial branches. The acromial branch often anastomoses with the suprascapular and posterior circumflex humeral arteries.

E. TRUE   Though many texts suggest that there is rarely any branch from the third part of the subclavian this artery occurs in ⅔ of dissections and arises quite commonly from this region. In about ⅓ of cases the superficial cervical and dorsal scapular arteries arise together from the thyrocervical trunk as the transverse cervical artery.

3. THORAX

The joints of the thorax include the:-

A. manubriosternal joint which is synovial
B. costochondral joints which are synovial
C. costovertebral joints which are supplied by ventral rami
D. 12th costotransverse joint
E. xiphisternal joint which often ossifies in old age.

Answers overleaf

TH1 Answers

A. FALSE This is a fibrocartilaginous or secondary cartilaginous joint which may become ossified. Most of the fibrocartilaginous joints are midline structures such as the pubic symphysis and intervertebral discs.

B. FALSE These are the hyaline cartilaginous joints between the costal cartilages and the small depressions in the ends of the shafts of each rib.

C. FALSE The costovertebral joints include the articulations of the heads of the ribs as well as the costotransverse joints between the tubercle of the rib and transverse process of the corresponding vertebra. Both joints are supplied by the thoracic dorsal rami.

D. FALSE The eleventh and twelfth ribs lack tubercles and have therefore no costotransverse joints.

E. TRUE

In the formation of the diaphragm:-

A. the pleuro-peritoneal membrane is the major contributor to the central tendon
B. the only motor supply is via C3,4,5
C. the sole sensory supply is the phrenic nerve
D. the right crus is shorter than the left
E. the aortic opening lies at the level of T12 and usually transmits the sympathetic chain.

Answers overleaf

TH2 Answers

   A.   FALSE   The development of the diaphragm is complex. In essence, however, the major contribution to the central tendon formation is from the septum transversum whilst the dorsolateral portion of the diaphragm is from the pleuro-peritoneal membrane, and the costal portion from the thoracic wall itself. A small region between the oesophagus and the aorta is formed by the dorsal mesentery.

   B.   TRUE   The phrenic nerve C3,4,5 is the only motor supply to the diaphragm. Each nerve supplies its respective side.

   C.   FALSE   The sensory supply is slightly more complex. The central portion of each dome is supplied via the phrenic nerve. Hence the classical referred pain to the C4 dermatome of the shoulder. However, there is also a segmental sensory supply to the peripheral part of the muscle via the lower six or seven intercostal nerves. Remember the diaphragm originates from slips of the lower six costal cartilages and ribs which interdigitate with the transversus abdominis muscle.

   D.   FALSE   The right crus, which originates from the bodies and intervertebral discs of L1,2,3 is both wider and longer than the left. It is through the medial fibres of the right crus that the oesophagus enters the abdomen bringing with it the vagal trunks, and oesophageal branches of the left gastric vessels.

   E.   FALSE   The aortic opening does indeed lie at the level of the lower border of T12 but it does not transmit the sympathetic chain. The ganglionated sympathetic chain usually enters the abdomen deep to the medial arcuate ligament or arch, lying on the psoas major muscle.

The thoracic duct:-

A. lies anterior to the internal jugular vein
B. lies posterior to the suprascapular artery
C. is anterior to the phrenic nerve at the level of C7
D. crosses anterior to the oesophagus at about the T4 level
E. is posterior to the posterior intercostal arteries.

TH4 Questions

Looking at a lateral view of a normal barium swallow you will notice that the:-

A. anterior wall is indented superiorly by the aortic arch
B. inferior portion of the anterior wall is indented by the right atrium
C. anterior wall is indented by the left main bronchus
D. descending thoracic aorta enters the abdomen at the T10 vertebral level
E. oesophagus enters the abdomen through the diaphragm at the T8 vertebral level.

Answers overleaf

35

TH3 Answers

A. & B. FALSE   The thoracic duct in the neck lies anterior to the arterial plane consisting of the subclavian artery and its branches, viz. vertebral, inferior thyroid, transverse cervical and suprascapular. However, it normally lies posterior to the three structures within the carotid sheath, i.e., internal jugular vein, carotid artery and vagus nerve.

C. TRUE   In the neck a useful landmark for the phrenic nerve is where it descends nearly vertically across scalenus anterior muscle. Here it is pinned down by the transverse cervical and suprascapular arteries.

D. FALSE   The thoracic duct most often lies to the right of the oesophagus in the thorax and at a level between T6 and T4 crosses posteriorly to the oesophagus.

E. FALSE   In the posterior mediastinum the thoracic duct, azygos vein and sympathetic chain all lie anterior to the posterior intercostal arteries. It is postulated that the horizontal structures belong to the thoracic wall itself and pass deep to longitudinal structures such as the thoracic duct.

TH4 Answers

A. B. & C.   TRUE, FALSE and TRUE   The oesophagus descends in the posterior mediastinum along the right side of the descending thoracic aorta, having passed behind and to the right of the aortic arch. The three indentations of the anterior wall of the oesophagus are caused by: superiorly the arch of the aorta, then the left main bronchus and inferiorly, the left atrium. It is this fact that is used in suspected cases of mitral stenosis when the left atrium enlarges and causes oesophageal constriction.

D. & E. FALSE   The three major structures to pierce the diaphragm are the inferior vena cava, oesophagus and aorta. The i.v.c. pierces the central tendon at the level of T 8 vertebra. It must, of course, pass through the tendon and not muscle fibres, otherwise one might faint 18 times a minute due to venous pooling! The oesophagus pierces the fibres of the right crus at the level of T 10, and is usually accompanied by the vagal trunks and left gastric vessels. The thoracic aorta leaves the chest deep to the fibrous arcuate ligament—one of the origins of the diaphragm itself—at the level of T 12 vertebra. It is therefore more correctly posterior to the diaphragm and does not truly pierce it (see T 2).

During an acute asthmatic attack a patient is sitting down with her hands grasping the arms of the chair for extra assistance. In this position during the inspiratory phase she will need the normal functions of the:-

A. lateral crico-arytenoid muscles
B. long thoracic nerves
C. latissimus dorsi muscles
D. spinal accessory nerves
E. scalenus anterior muscles.

Answers overleaf

TH5 Answers

A. FALSE In laboured breathing associated with acute respiratory distress the nostrils and glottis dilate rhythmically, allowing easier passage of air. In the larynx the lateral crico-arytenoid is often inseparable from the thyro-arytenoid and on contraction it draws the muscular process of the arytenoid forwards. This rotates the vocal cord medially, resulting in closure of the rima glottidis as in phonation. In acute respiratory disease the cords must be opened and it is the posterior crico-arytenoid which performs this function. Arising from the cricoid it is inserted into the muscular process of the arytenoid. On contraction it rotates the vocal process laterally, resulting in the opening of the rima glottidis. It is, in fact, the only abductor of the vocal folds as a whole.

B. TRUE The long thoracic nerve (Bell) originates directly from the roots of C5,6, 7 and supplies the eight slips of serratus anterior muscle. This muscle is important in asthma cases as it helps in fixation of the scapula and hence gives a firm platform for muscles such as pectoralis major and minor to elevate the ribs.

C. FALSE Latissimus dorsi is used in deep expiration, not inspiration. It is particularly evident in a short sharp explosive expiration such as a cough.

D. TRUE On two accounts, as this nerve supplies both trapezius and sternomastoid muscles. The trapezius is used in fixation of the scapulae (see B) and the medial head of the sternomastoid raises the manubrium at the end of each inspiration.

E. TRUE The scalene muscles raise the first and second ribs and work in tandem with the sternomastoid to raise the upper rib cage and increase the antero-posterior diameter in the superior mediastinum.

In the superior mediastinum:-

A. the cardiac plexus lies anterior to the bifurcation of the trachea
B. the highest intercostal artery lies on the neck of the first rib
C. the left phrenic nerve lies anterior to the brachiocephalic vein
D. the left superior intercostal vein lies between the vagus posteriorly and the phrenic anteriorly
E. the right phrenic nerve runs subpleurally along the pericardium overlying the right atrium.

Answers overleaf

A. TRUE   The cardiac plexus is a mixed plexus of sympathetic fibres from the upper four thoracic levels, and cervical ganglia, and parasympathetic fibres from the vagus. Sometimes it is further subdivided into pulmonary and aortic plexus.

B. TRUE   This artery which usually arises from the costocervical trunk is the odd man out in the arterial supply to the intercostal spaces. After descending anterior to the neck of the first rib with the sympathetic trunk medially, it gives off the first posterior intercostal artery, then continues in front of the second rib becoming the second posterior intercostal artery. The course of these two posterior intercostals is similar to the remaining nine which arise from the back of the aorta itself.

C. FALSE   The key to the relative positions in this region is to remember that the phrenic nerve lies on the scalenus anterior muscle. This muscle divides the subclavian vein anteriorly from its artery which lies with the trunks of the brachial plexus posterior to the muscle. The brachiocephalic vein is anterior to the nerves and main arteries of the neck. In childhood its upper border may rise above the suprasternal notch and be in danger during tracheostomy.

D. TRUE   A useful landmark for difficult vivas, the left superior intercostal vein is formed by the second, third and sometimes the fourth posterior intercostal veins. It passes up over the arch of the aorta and enters the left brachiocephalic vein just at the point where the phrenic nerve changes from being lateral to the vagus to being anterior. It is here that the left superior intercostal vein separates the two nerves.

E. TRUE   The right phrenic nerve enters the thorax posterior to the internal jugular and descends subpleurally along the 'great venous channel line', viz., superior vena cava, the right atrium and the inferior vena cava.

In the adult human heart:-

A. the pericardium consists of three layers
B. the sulcus terminalis is often seen in the right atrium
C. musculi pectinati develop from the primitive sinus venosus
D. the intraventricular septum is entirely fleshy
E. the oblique sinus is an immediate anterior relation of the oesophagus.

Answers overleaf

41

TH7 Answers

A. TRUE   The pericardium consists of an outer tough fibrous sac, lined by an inner serous sac. During development the heart and roots of the great vessels invaginate the serous sac from behind. Consequently the serous pericardium has both a parietal and visceral layer. The visceral layer is also known as the epicardium. It is the potential space between these two layers (pericardial cavity) that fills with fluid in pericarditis requiring aspiration.

B. & C. FALSE   The sulcus terminalis is never seen in the right atrium but often on its exterior. It is the crista terminalis that is inside the right atrium. This is a ridge of muscle indicating where the primitive atrium and sinus venosus have merged during development. In the right atrium the portion behind the crista terminalis is smooth as it has developed from the sinus venosus. The anterior portion is trabeculated as it developed from the primitive atrium. These trabeculations or musculi pectinati (pecten Latin = comb) can also be seen in both auricular appendages.

D. FALSE   Though mostly fleshy, the interventricular septum has a thin membranous region in its uppermost border about the size of a penny piece. The fleshy part is an upgrowth from the apex, the membranous part is a downgrowth from the interatrial septum. Failure of these two parts to meet may result in an interventricular septal defect (v.s.d.) with a shunt from the high pressured left to lower pressured right ventricle

E. TRUE   The reflection of pericardium at the veins leaves an irregular line around a space termed the oblique sinus of the pericardium. It is limited on the sides by the right and left pulmonary veins as well as the inferior vena cava on the right. It is behind the left atrium and in front of the oesophagus (see TH4).

The blood supply of the normal adult heart includes the:-

A. anterior interventricular branch of the right coronary artery which descends to the apical region

B. right coronary artery which gives off the sinus node artery

C. anterior cardiac veins which drain into the coronary sinus

D. venae cordis minimae or Thebesian veins which open into the left atrium

E. coronary sinus which collects blood from the great and middle cardiac veins.

Answers overleaf

TH8 Answers

A. FALSE The anterior interventricular artery is a major branch of the left coronary artery, the other being the circumflex branch. It is this artery, accompanied by the great cardiac vein, which is very obvious on examination of a dissected heart. It lies in the intraventricular groove on the anterior surface of the heart, though it is often obscured by fat deposits.

B. TRUE

C. D. & E. FALSE, TRUE and TRUE The heart is drained partly by veins that empty into the coronary sinus and partly by small veins that empty directly into the chambers of the heart. These small veins include the anterior cardiac veins which drain the anterior part of the right ventricle, cross the coronary (atrio-ventricular) groove and end directly in the right atrium. The venae cordis minimae are tiny veins in the heart substance which end directly into the nearest cavity, though mainly into the two atria. The major venous drainage vessel is the coronary sinus which develops from the left horn of the sinus venosus. It is about 4 çm long and lies in the atrio-ventricular groove posteriorly opening into the right atrium. Its tributaries include the great cardiac vein, the posterior vein of the left ventricle, the middle cardiac vein and the small cardiac vein. The oblique vein of the left atrium, which is the remains of the embryonic left common cardiac vein, also drains into the coronary sinus.

A cachectic elderly man with obvious chest problems enters your clinic. On initial X-ray examination he is thought to have a carcinoma of the right lung arising in the apex. On closer physical examination you might expect to find:-

A. dilatation of the right pupil
B. paralysis of the right levator palpebrae superioris muscle
C. a sweating right palm
D. pain and tingling in the region of the right index finger
E. wasting of the interossei of the right hand.

Useful surface markings in the chest include the:-

A. right nipple (of the non-pendulous breast) as the extreme limit of the upper border of the liver
B. second thoracic vertebra as the level at which the trachea bifurcates
C. suprasternal (jugular) notch as the level of the second thoracic vertebra
D. xiphisternal joint as the level of the disc between the ninth and tenth thoracic vertebrae
E. first prominent bony bump when palpating the spine from above downwards as the first thoracic spine.

Answers overleaf

TH9 Answers

A. & B. FALSE and TRUE   An apical carcinoma of the lung often invades locally and thus affects the sympathetic chain, upper ribs and at a later stage the lower trunks of the brachial plexus. These tumours are often referred to as Pancoast tumours (American radiologist of early 20th century). The effects of pressure on the sympathetic chain often leads to a Horner's syndrome (Swiss ophthalmologist of 19th century) where one may see a partial drooping of the eyelid (ptosis) due to paralysis of about one third of the levator palpebrae superioris, the rest being innervated by the third cranial nerve; and a constricted pupil due to unopposed parasympathetic action of the constrictor pupillae. Dilation of the pupil with a drooped eyelid is seen in third nerve lesions.

C. FALSE   Absence of sweating (anhidrosis) is also seen in Horner's syndrome and this often extends down the arm to the palm so that the hand of the affected side is dry.

D. FALSE   The lower trunk of the brachial plexus (C8, T1) is invaded as it crosses the first rib posterior to the subclavian artery and so the distribution of pain and tingling tends to be in the cutaneous distribution of the ulnar nerve, i.e. the little finger side of the hand.

E. TRUE   If the lower brachial plexus lesion was of long enough standing the muscles supplied by the ulnar nerve, such as the interossei or hypothenar muscles, may show wasting.

TH10 Answers

A. TRUE   This is of course also the surface marking for the right dome of the diaphragm. The left dome or cupola is usually 2 – 3 cm below the left nipple.

B. FALSE   Bifurcation occurs at or below the sternal angle of Louis and slightly to the right. This level is classically at T4 but it must be realised that the bifurcation is not fixed and moves downwards some 2 – 3 cm in the erect breathing individual.

C. TRUE

D. TRUE

E. FALSE   Usually the first bump is the 7th cervical process (vertebra prominens) and in many subjects two obvious spines of C7 and T1 are visible as well as palpable. T1—T4 are easily felt and usually seen. T6—T12 are much harder to distinguish.

4. ABDOMEN

Peritoneal folds which contain an artery and a vein include the:-

A. median umbilical fold
B. falciform ligament
C. lienorenal ligament
D. lateral umbilical fold
E. medial umbilical fold.

Answers overleaf

ABD1 Answers

A. FALSE   The median umbilical ligament is a remnant of the urachus and extends from the apex of the bladder to the umbilicus. The part nearest to the bladder usually retains its lumen which may communicate with that of the bladder. The degenerating allantois is continuous, at the umbilicus, with the urachus. The median umbilical ligament raises a fold of peritoneum called the median umbilical fold.

B. FALSE   The falciform ligament develops from the ventral mesogastrium and in the adult joins the liver to the anterior body wall. It is one of the six folds of peritoneum converging on the umbilicus and contains in its free border the ligamentum teres, which is the obliterated remnant of the left umbilical vein. It also often contains what is called the anterior abdominal fat body.

C. TRUE   The lienorenal ligament connects the spleen to the kidney and posterior abdominal wall. It transmits the splenic vessels and the tail of the pancreas.

D. TRUE   The lateral umbilical folds contain the inferior epigastric vessels which extend from the medial border of the deep inguinal ring to the arcuate line of the posterior rectus sheath.

E. FALSE   The medial umbilical ligament contains the obliterated umbilical artery which is usually seen in the adult as the first visceral branch of the internal iliac. In the fetus the two umbilical arteries are the main channels from the aorta to the placenta. After delivery the distal portion of the artery atrophies. The cord-like fibrous remnant from the pelvis to the umbilicus is covered by peritoneum and is called the medial umbilical fold.

A daring young lady has a tattoo drawn as a complete circle around her umbilicus. She is unlucky and develops infection in both superficial and deeper tissues. You might expect her to have tender nodes in the:-

A. left central axillary group
B. right superficial inguinal group
C. right internal thoracic group
D. left external iliac group
E. 10th intercostal space.

The ureter:-

A. is the immediate anterior relation of the transverse processes of the third and fourth lumbar vertebrae
B. can, on vaginal examination, be palpated in the posterior fornix
C. on the right is an anterior relation of the duodenum
D. lies anterior to the genitofemoral nerve but posterior to the gonadal vessels
E. drains to the lateral aortic lymph nodes.

Answers overleaf

ABD2 Answers

A. & B. TRUE   The skin of the abdominal wall is drained by lymph vessels that radiate from the umbilicus. It is as if you have tied a belt around the waist at this level and all the skin above drains to the axillary lymph nodes; all the skin and superficial tissues below the belt drain to the superficial inguinal lymph nodes (see PEL2). In this case, as her tattoo is a total para-umbilical circle, both axillary and superficial inguinal nodes will be involved.

C. & D. TRUE   As she has deeper infection (into the rectus sheath) it is likely that the lymphatics accompanying the superior and inferior epigastric vessels will carry this infection to the internal thoracic and external iliac nodes respectively.

E. FALSE   There are rarely any lymph nodes in the intercostal spaces, only vessels leading into the posterior mediastinum or abdominal wall. You may have been misled by remembering that the cutaneous nerve supply to the umbilicus is the tenth thoracic nerve.

ABD3 Answers

A. FALSE   Though always easy to remember, especially from radiographs, that it lies anterior to the tips of the transverse processes of L2, 3, 4, 5, it is not their immediate anterior relation. The medial edge of the psoas major muscle separates the two.

B. FALSE   In the female the ureter passes just above the lateral fornix of the vagina, and here lies below the broad ligament and uterine vessels. It is here that a diseased ureter or one containing a stone might be palpated.

C. FALSE   It is the descending (second) part of the duodenum which lies anterior to the beginning of the right ureter.

D. TRUE   The way to remember the order of structures on the posterior abdominal wall and pelvic brim is that the alimentary system is anterior to the genital, urinary and posterior abdominal wall structures in that order respectively.

E. TRUE   Lymphatics from the kidney and upper ureter drain to the lateral aortic nodes. From the lower abdominal ureter the drainage is to the common iliac group and the pelvic ureter drains to the internal iliac nodes.

You are asked to perform a percutaneous liver biopsy through the ninth right intercostal space in the mid-axillary line. Pondering on the procedure you are about to perform, you reason that the structures your needle normally pierces include the:-

A. costodiaphragmatic recess
B. pleural cavity
C. diaphragm
D. serratus anterior muscle
E. external oblique muscle.

Your patient is admitted with portal hypertension due to his drinking habits. Knowing how bloody it is to operate on regions of porto-systemic venous anastomosis in this kind of patient you would be loath to operate on the:-

A. upper oesophagus
B. recto-sigmoid junction
C. umbilicus
D. descending mesocolon
E. extraperitoneal portion of the liver.

Answers overleaf

ABD4 Answers

A. B. & C. TRUE   This site, through an intercostal space, is the most commonly used for liver biopsy, although in patients with enlarged livers a biopsy may be more easily performed through the anterior abdominal wall below the costal margin. Having decided on the exact intercostal space by examination and, especially, percussion the needle is introduced closely above the rib in order to avoid the neuro-vascular bundle which grooves the inferior border of each rib. The needle passes through the superficial fascia and fibres of external oblique muscle before entering the intercostal muscles. It then pierces the costo-parietal pleura which descends usually as far as the 10th rib in the mid-axillary line. The pleura is then reflected from the ribs on to the diaphragm. The lower border of the lung does not extend so far inferiorly as this reflexion, the gap being the costodiaphragmatic recess. This is of course just a named part of the pleural cavity. Having crossed this recess the needle pierces the diaphragmatic pleura and diaphragm.

D. FALSE   Serratus anterior arises by eight muscular slips from the upper eight ribs and costal cartilages.

E. TRUE   (See A above).

ABD5 Answers

A. & B. FALSE   The sites of porto-systemic venous anastomosis do include the oesophagus and rectum, but the lowest end of both, rather than their most proximal portion. In the oesophagus it is branches of the left gastric vein and the lower azygos vein system which dilate to cause varices and later haematemeses. In the rectum anastomosis occurs between the superior haemorrhoidal branch of the inferior mesenteric vein (portal) and the inferior haemorrhoidal veins draining to the internal iliac veins (systemic).

C. TRUE   The veins of the superior and inferior epigastric system (systemic) anastomose with veins running along the falciform ligament to the umbilicus. Dilatation of these venous channels will cause a 'caput Medusae' radiating from the umbilicus.

D. TRUE   There are portal tributaries in the mesentery, and in the mesocolon, particularly of the ascending and descending colon, and these tributaries anastomose with the systemic veins of the posterior abdominal wall, i.e. the lumbar, renal and, more superiorly, the phrenic.

E. TRUE   This is of course the 'bare area' and it is here that portal branches in the liver communicate with the systemic veins of the diaphragm.

During laparotomy you deliver two lengths of small intestine. You would be able to distinguish the ileum from jejunum because, comparing the two, the ileum has:-

A. thicker walls than the jejunum
B. less valvulae conniventes
C. appendices epiploicae and occasionally taeniae coli
D. less fat overlying the mesentery
E. fewer arterial arcades and shorter terminal vessels.

The structures on which the stomach lies are often referred to as the 'stomach bed'. *Immediate* posterior relations of the stomach wall include the:-

A. lesser sac of the peritoneum
B. pancreas
C. splenic artery
D. gastric surface of the spleen
E. duodenojejunal flexure.

Answers overleaf

ABD6 Answers

A. & B. FALSE and TRUE   The small intestine is some 4 – 8 metres long; the upper half is called the jejunum and the rest the ileum. There is no sharp distinction between the two but as one traces the bowel distally certain changes in character do appear. The jejunum is thicker walled due to the presence of the larger circular folds in the mucous membrane (valvulae conniventes or plicae circulares). These are particularly easy to see on a double air contrast, opaque meal small bowel x-ray.

C. FALSE   An obvious trick. The small bowel can be distinguished from large bowel by these two features. The appendices epiploicae are small numerous fat-laden peritoneal tags seen over most of the large bowel save the appendix, caecum and rectum. The taeniae coli are flattened bands of longitudinal muscle involved in peristalsis; these are not seen on the appendix or rectum. It is these bands that cause the characteristic sacculations or haustrations of the large bowel.

D. FALSE   The mesentery carries more fat distally.

E. FALSE   It is true that the ileum does have shorter terminal vessels but that is because of the greater number of arcades in the ileum. Remember the ileum has more fat, and more arcades but is thinner walled and smaller in diameter than the jejunum.

ABD7 Answers

A. B. & C. TRUE, FALSE and FALSE   The lesser sac is indeed the true *immediate* posterior relation of the stomach, separating it from the pancreas, left kidney, adrenal gland, splenic artery, left colic flexure and the upper layer of the transverse mesocolon.

D. FALSE   The gastric surface of the spleen is generally referred to as part of the stomach bed but in fact it is separated from the posterior wall of the stomach by an intervening layer of the greater sac of peritoneum.

E. FALSE   The greater omentum and the transverse mesocolon separate the stomach from the duodenojejunal flexure and the small intestine.
It is worth noting that although not *immediate* posterior relations of the stomach, all the previously mentioned structures including the diaphragm are directly posterior to the stomach and may be involved in clinical situations.

A patient is admitted to your hospital experiencing pain in both the right hypochondrium and the right scapular region. Apart from upper abdominal tenderness, physical examination is negative and laboratory tests of hepatic function are normal. You might suggest there is a stone in the:-

A. common hepatic duct
B. right kidney
C. cystic duct
D. gallbladder
E. duodenal papilla.

The tenth thoracic nerve supplies the:-

A. kidney
B. testes
C. appendix
D. diaphragm
E. suprapubic skin.

Answers overleaf

55

ABD8 Answers

A. FALSE   If your patient really did have a stone blocking the common hepatic duct, it would most likely reveal itself as a jaundiced patient and cause some abnormality in the laboratory tests.

B. FALSE   A stone in the right kidney might indeed cause acute upper abdominal pain without abnormal laboratory tests of hepatic function. However, the patient would be most unlikely to have shoulder pain, for the nerves which supply the kidney are derived from the tenth, eleventh and twelfth thoracic segments of the spinal cord. Referred pain from a renal lesion would therefore be in these dermatomes.

C. & D. TRUE   Referred pain to the shoulder is a classical presentation of gallbladder disease. Normal hepatic function is compatible with a stone blocking either the neck of the gallbladder or the cystic duct, since neither lesions necessarily interferes with drainage of bile from the liver. The nerves of the gallbladder, which are mainly sympathetic, are derived from the coeliac plexus and travel along the hepatic artery and its branches.

E. FALSE   For similar reasons as in A, the patient would have abnormal liver function tests.

ABD9 Answers

A. TRUE   The nerves of the kidney, although small, are about fifteen in number and are derived from T10, T11 and T12 (see ABD 8B).

B. & C. TRUE   Testes and ovaries, as well as the mid-gut including the appendix, are probably supplied by T10. The sensory supply of the T10 dermatome is to the umbilical region and this is easily shown by watching the effects on a rugby player who is kicked in the crutch with bruising of the testes. The referred testicular pain is in the para-umbilical region as is the pain of ovulation. An early appendicitis also illustrates this point well as the initial pain is para-umbilical and only moves to the right iliac fossa when the local parietal peritoneum is involved.

D. TRUE   The sensory supply to the periphery of the diaphragm is from the lower five intercostal nerves. The motor supply is from the phrenic nerve only.

E. FALSE   (See B and C). The skin of the suprapubic region is supplied by branches of T12 and L1.

The inguinal canal:-

A. transmits the ilioinguinal nerve in men only
B. transmits the genital branch of the genito-femoral nerve in both sexes
C. in the newborn is more oblique than in the adult
D. has the fascia transversalis and conjoint tendon along its posterior wall
E. has the external oblique muscle as its roof.

Answers overleaf

ABD10 Answers

  A. FALSE   The ilioinguinal nerve (L1) is transmitted in both sexes. In the male the contents of the spermatic cord are also transmitted whereas in the female the ilioinguinal nerve, genital branch of the genito-femoral nerve and the round ligament of the uterus pass along the canal. Accompanying the round ligament are lymphatics (see PEL 2).

  B. TRUE   In the male the genital branch of this nerve is involved in the cremaster reflex, but as the female has no such muscle it is perhaps surprising that this branch of the nerve passes along the canal to end in the labium majus and skin of the mons pubis.

  C. FALSE   In the newborn the deep ring lies almost directly behind the superficial so the canal is both shorter and less oblique than in the adult. During growth the deep ring moves laterally to form a more oblique canal, usually about 4 cm. long in the adult.

  D. TRUE   The inguinal canal has the fascia transversalis along its entire posterior wall. In the medial third this is reinforced by the conjoint tendon which is the final common tendon of the internal oblique and transversus abdominis muscles. This tough tendon inserts into the pubic crest and pectineal line and therefore forms a tough posterior wall behind the sole defect in the external oblique muscle, the superficial inguinal ring.

  E. FALSE   The roof of the canal is formed by the arching fibres of internal oblique and transversus muscles (see D). The aponeurosis of the external oblique muscle is the entire anterior wall, reinforced laterally by fibres of internal oblique originating from the inguinal ligament.

58

5. PELVIS

The pelvic splanchnic nerve:-

A. crosses the ischial spine medial to the pudendal artery
B. contains postganglionic parasympathetic visceral motor fibres
C. arises from the posterior primary rami of S2, 3 and 4
D. supplies motor fibres to the sigmoid colon
E. produces erection of the penis.

Answers overleaf

PEL1 Answers

A. B. & C. FALSE   A common mistake is to confuse the pelvic splanchnic nerve with the pudendal nerve. Both nerves originate from the anterior primary rami of S2, 3, 4 and occasionally S5. The pelvic splanchnic nerve contains preganglionic parasympathetic fibres on their way via the inferior hypogastric plexus to the various pelvic viscera. The pudendal nerve, however, contains motor, sensory and postganglionic sympathetic fibres. It leaves the pelvis through the greater sciatic foramen below piriformis, crosses the ischial spine medial to the pudendal artery and then enters the perineum through the lesser sciatic foramen. After passing along the pudendal canal (Alcock) in the lateral wall of the ischio-rectal fossa it gives off its branches, i.e. inferior rectal nerve, perineal nerve and dorsal nerve of the penis (clitoris).

D. TRUE   The preganglionic parasympathetic fibres which reach the inferior hypogastric (pelvic) plexus, on either side, supply the descending colon, sigmoid colon and the pelvic viscera.

E. TRUE   The pelvic splanchnic nerves cause relaxation of the arteries to the pudendal erectile tissue, producing erection of the penis or clitoris, hence the alternative name 'nervi erigentes'. They also carry afferent fibres from the pelvis, especially pain and distension.

A woman complains of tender hard swellings in the groin. On examination they are correctly diagnosed as superficial inguinal lymph nodes. To find the cause of this swelling one would need to examine the:-

A. anal canal above the pectinate line
B. the body of the uterus
C. lateral portion of the uterine tubes
D. vagina
E. skin overlying the calf muscles.

Answers overleaf

PEL2 Answers

A. FALSE   The anal canal is the terminal 3 – 4 cm of the gastro-intestinal tract and is a transition zone between the embryonic proctodeum (ectoderm) and the cloaca (endoderm). The line of demarcation is known as the 'pecten' or pectinate line and is characterised by the anal valves (Ball) which lie at the distal end of the numerous vertical folds of mucous membrane called the anal columns (Morgagni). The pectinate line is thus an important developmental landmark, superiorly the epithelium changes from squamous to columnar and the pale pink skin gives way to plum-coloured mucosa. The blood supply differs also, the superior haemorrhoidal artery (a branch of the inferior mesenteric) supplies above the line and the inferior haemorrhoidal artery (a branch of the internal iliac) below it. The corresponding veins and lymphatics are also divided in a similar manner, above the line draining to the internal iliac nodes and below the pectinate line to the superficial inguinal nodes.

B. TRUE   Though most of the uterus drains via vessels in the broad ligament to the external and common iliac nodes there is a small region of the fundus which drains to the superomedial group of superficial inguinal nodes. This drainage is via a single vessel running along the round ligament of the uterus to the mons pubis. Development of the guberaculum ovarii helps explain this course of drainage (ref.   ).

C. FALSE   The uterine (Fallopian) tubes drain with the vessels of the ovary to the pre-aortic and lateral aortic nodes. They transverse the broad ligament and cross the pelvic brim ending in nodes between the renal vessels above, and the common iliac vessels below.

D. TRUE   The upper portion of the vagina drains to the external iliac, internal iliac and, via vessels passing in the utero-sacral fold, to the lateral sacral lymph nodes and others found on the sacral promontory. The lower end of the vagina, however, like the anus below the pectinate line, and the labium majus drain to the superficial inguinal nodes.

E. FALSE   The superficial inguinal nodes receive nearly all the superficial lymph vessels of the lower limb. There is one exception and that is the region drained via the short saphenous vein, i.e. the skin of the lateral dorsum of the foot and skin overlying the calf muscles. This region drains via the popliteal nodes in the popliteal fossa and hence to the deep lymphatic system.

62

Male/female homologous structures are:-

A. bulbo-urethral glands   — greater vestibular glands
B. duct of the epididymis — duct of the epoöphoron
C. gubernaculum testis   — ligament of the ovary
D. prostatic gland   — greater vestibular gland
E. penis   — clitoris.

Answers overleaf

PEL3 Answers

A. TRUE   The bulbo-urethral glands (Cowper) which lie within the deep perineal pouch are surrounded by the sphincter urethrae muscle fibres. In the female the greater vestibular glands (Bartholin) open into the posterior portion of the vestibule via a 2 cm duct.

B. TRUE   The duct of the epididymis and the efferent ductules of the testes correspond to the epoöphoron which is a vestigial part of the mesonephric duct in the female.

C. TRUE   The gubernaculum testis (helmsman) is homologous with the gubernaculum ovarii which becomes both the ligament of the ovary and the round ligament of the uterus. The former attaches the ovary to the uterus whereas the round ligament follows the course of the spermatic cord into the inguinal canal and ends in the mons pubis just medial to the superficial inguinal ring.

D. FALSE   The prostatic gland has no true homologue in the female but many believe that the para-urethral glands and their ducts which open on each side of the female urethra are the most likely homologous structures. These are called the ducts of Skene and they are prone to infection, especially with the gonococcus.

E. TRUE   Both of these structures form from the undifferentiated genital tubercle.

The ischiorectal fossa:-

A. is bounded medially by the rectum
B. is bounded laterally by the fascia of obturator internus muscle
C. extends deep to the perineal membrane in the urogenital triangle
D. contains structures which have emerged from the pelvis through the lesser sciatic foramen
E. is roofed by the fascia of levator ani muscle.

In the pelvis the:-

A. sacral hiatus permits entrance into the epidural space
B. rectum follows the sacral concavity
C. sacral promontory is palpable on rectal examination
D. sacrotuberous ligament divides the greater from the lesser sciatic foramen
E. levator ani muscle originates from the pelvic fascia overlying the obturator internus muscle.

Answers overleaf

PEL4 Answers

A. & B. FALSE and TRUE Contrary to its name the two ischiorectal fossae do not border on the rectum but only the anal sphincter muscles. The external anal sphincter is reinforced by the levator ani muscle and this forms the superomedial aspect of the fossae. Laterally the fascia covering the obturator internus forms a boundary. Contained in this wall is a fascial tunnel (Alcock's canal) whose contents include the internal pudendal vessels and pudendal nerve (see D below). It is worth noting that the obturator internus muscle lies on the ischium but the ischium itself is not an immediate lateral relation, save possibly the tuberosity.

C. TRUE It is also important to realize that these fossae communicate with each other posterior to the anus and so infection in one may rapidly spread to the other. The partial separation of the two fossae is by the anococcygeal body, a fibrous septum between anus and coccyx.

D. FALSE The structures that emerge from the lesser sciatic foramen are the tendon of obturator internus and its accompanying gemelli muscles. The trick in this question is that the pudendal vessels leave the greater sciatic foramen, hook over the ischial spine (a useful bony landmark for pudendal blocks) and then enter the perineum via the lesser sciatic foramen (see PEL 1).

E. TRUE

PEL5 Answers

A. TRUE This is the site of the caudal epidural block often performed in obstetrics.

B. TRUE

C. FALSE The sacral promontory is at the proximal rectum and not within reach of the examining finger in the rectum. You may have confused this with the fact that in thin women the promontory is palpable on vaginal examination in a narrow pelvis.

D. FALSE It is the sacrospinous ligament that divides up the foramina.

E. TRUE Levator ani originates from a tendinous arch (white line) which arches over the obturator internus fascia. It also has origins from the body of the pelvis, and the ischial spine.

A radiologist shows you an excellent selective internal iliac arteriogram. You notice that of the numerous branches, those derived from its anterior trunk include the:-

A. artery to the sciatic nerve
B. superior gluteal artery
C. inferior epigastric artery—pubic branch
D. artery to the vas deferens
E. uterine artery.

PEL7 Questions

You are finding difficulty in passing a urinary catheter in an elderly male patient; the catheter seems to stick at certain points. The likely sites for this to happen are at the narrowest parts of the urethra which are:-

A. the navicular fossa
B. at the site of the colliculus seminalis (verumontanum)
C. at the level of the perineal membrane
D. the internal urethral orifice
E. the external urethral orifice.

Answers overleaf

PEL6 Answers

A. TRUE   The largest terminal branch of the anterior trunk of the internal iliac artery is the inferior gluteal artery. Leaving the greater sciatic foramen it passes into the gluteal region and descends the leg in company with the sciatic nerve lying deep to gluteus maximus. The artery to the sciatic nerve is a long slender branch of the inferior gluteal.

B. FALSE   This is the largest branch of the internal iliac and the termination of its posterior trunk.

C. FALSE   The inferior epigastric artery is a branch of the external iliac arising just above the inguinal ligament. The pubic branch descends close to the femoral ring behind the pubis and anastomoses with the pubic branch of the obturator. In 20 – 30% of people this branch replaces the obturator artery and occasionally its course goes along the free edge of the lacunar ligament. In these cases it is liable to damage during femoral herniae repairs.

D. TRUE   This is a branch of the superior vesicular artery and it often anastomoses with the testicular artery around the testes. Occasionally the artery to the vas is from another branch of the anterior trunk—the inferior vesicular artery.

E. TRUE

PEL7 Answers

A. FALSE   The navicular fossa is a dilatation just inside the very narrow external urethral orifice.

B. FALSE   The colliculus seminalis (or verumontanum) is the summit of the urethral crest and is situated in the prostatic urethra. This portion of the urethra is about 3 cm long and is the widest and most dilatable region.

C. TRUE   The perineal membrane is the lowest border of the narrowest part of the urethra, the membranous part. This section is only 2 cm long and is very firmly anchored by the membrane. It is here that problems are often encountered for not only is the membrane itself an obstacle but immediately deep to it is the sphincter urethrae.

D. FALSE   This is a wide open canal from the bladder into the prostatic urethra, although it functions as an involuntary sphincter.

E. TRUE   The male urethra is approximately 20 cm long and the narrowest part is the external orifice.

The deep perineal pouch:-

A. is limited by the superficial perineal fascia and the perineal membrane
B. contains the bulbourethral glands and the openings of their ducts
C. contains the narrow membranous urethra
D. contains the sphincter urethrae and deep transverse perineal muscles
E. transmits the dorsal nerve of the penis.

On examination of an elderly male patient you find a swelling around the left testis which tracks up the left spermatic cord towards the external inguinal canal. It feels vascular in character and you therefore consider its pathogenesis might be:-

A. a renal vein thrombosis
B. a left inguinal hernia
C. an invasive renal carcinoma
D. a loaded sigmoid colon
E. inflammation of the parietal tunica vaginalis.

Answers overleaf

PEL8 Answers

A. FALSE This is a description of the boundaries of the superficial perineal pouch. The deep pouch is bounded by the perineal membrane inferiorly and the superior fascia of the urogenital diaphragm superiorly.

B. & C. FALSE and TRUE The two pea-sized bulbo-urethral glands of Cowper lie alongside the narrow membranous urethra, both lying in the deep perineal pouch. The ducts however travel in the wall of the urethra for a couple of centimetres before piercing the perineal membrane and opening into the spongy urethra. It is these glands and ducts that are infected in gonorrhoea (see PEL 3).

D. & E. TRUE The other contents of the deep perineal pouch consist of a sheet of muscle fibres comprising the sphincter and the transverse perineal muscles. Also passing through the deep pouch are nerves and vessels, branches of the internal pudendal artery and pudendal nerve. The dorsal nerve of the penis is one such nerve supplying the glands, prepuce, skin of the penis and spongy urethra.

PEL9 Answers

A. TRUE It should be obvious from the signs that one is dealing with a varicosity of the pampiniform plexus (varicocele). The left side is usually affected because the left testicular vein drains into the renal vein on the left and not into the IVC as occurs on the right.

B. TRUE After leaving the testis the pampiniform plexus, as part of the spermatic cord, enters the inguinal canal and might therefore be compressed by an inguinal hernia also in the canal.

C. TRUE One of the classical sites of spread for renal tumours is along the renal vein itself. This would of course block the entrance of the left testicular vein (see A).

D. TRUE As the sigmoid colon is an immediate anterior relation it also might cause pressure and obstruction of the venous return.

E. FALSE Do not confuse a varicocele with a hydrocele which is fluid between the visceral and parietal layers of the tunica vaginalis. It normally would feel very different and unless the processus vaginalis was still patent would not track towards the inguinal canal.

You deliver a woman of a 5 kg baby boy. Unfortunately an inadequate episiotomy was performed and a large posterior central tear resulted. Whilst sewing up this third degree tear, which went as far as the rectum, you reflect that the muscles which have been damaged include the:-

A. external anal sphincter
B. anterior fibres of both levatores ani
C. ischiocavernosus
D. deep transverse perineal muscles
E. superficial transverse perineal muscles.

Answers overleaf

A. & B. TRUE It should be obvious from the story that the woman has a damaged perineal body or 'central tendon' of the perineum though this region is not in fact tendinous. It lies some 1 – 2 cm anterior to the anus and just posterior to the introitus of the female or bulb of the penis in the male. It is an anchor point for eight muscles of the perineum where they meet, blend and interdigitate. These include the external anal sphincter, bulbospongiosus, the two transverse perinei, both superficial and deep, and some anterior fibres of the two levatores ani. In addition a few fibres are contributed from the rectal ampulla and anal canal. If the perineal body is not repaired properly the levator ani anterior fibres cause an enlarged gap in the pelvic floor during contraction. This may result in a cystocele or in more severe cases prolapse of the uterus or rectum.

C. FALSE Ischiocavernosus covers the crus clitoris and does not meet in the middle as does bulbospongiosus.

D. TRUE

E. TRUE

6. LOWER LIMB

A soldier is standing erect with a fully extended knee. One would expect that the:-

A. rectus femoris is contracted
B. oblique posterior ligament is relaxed
C. fibular collateral ligaments are taut
D. anterior cruciate ligament is taut
E. posterior parts of the menisci are compressed.

You notice that your patient has a dipping gait, the left side of his pelvis drooping when the right leg is supporting his body weight. Possible causes of this situation include damage to:-

A. the right sciatic nerve
B. the nerve roots L5, S1, 2 on the left
C. the nerve roots L4, 5 and S1 on the right
D. his right superior gluteal nerve
E. his left inferior gluteal nerve.

Answers overleaf

LL1 Answers

A. FALSE During the process of extension the rectus femoris and ligamentum patellae are tightened but once in the erect fully extended position the extensors are relaxed. Remember the position in which you examine a mobile patella.

B. C. & D. FALSE, TRUE and TRUE In the extended knee both cruciate ligaments, the fibular and tibial collateral ligaments, the posterior oblique ligament and capsule are all taut. The cruciate ligaments are fairly taut in all positions of the knee as their function is to prevent the tibia being carried too far forwards (anterior cruciate) or backwards (posterior cruciate) with respect to the femur.

E. FALSE It is in flexion, not extension, that the posterior portion of the menisci are compressed between femur and tibia.

LL2 Answers

A. FALSE The muscles that support the pelvis are the abductor muscle group of the supporting leg. In this case, where the right leg is on the ground, it is the abductors of the right side whose origin and insertion are exchanged in a functional sense. The abductors include gluteus medius, minimus and tensor fasciae latae. None of these muscles is supplied by the sciatic nerve.

B. FALSE The three abductors are all supplied by the superior gluteal nerve whose roots of origin are L4,5 and S1. As mentioned before, it would be a lesion of the right sided abductors which would cause the left side of the pelvis to droop.

C. & D. TRUE The right superior gluteal nerve has its roots of origin in L4,5 and S1. Damage to these roots or the right superior gluteal nerve itself would cause paralysis to the right abductors and hence the left side of the pelvis would be unable to rise up during its swing phase of walking.

E. FALSE This is wrong on two counts, firstly as explained above the lesion would be on the right, not the left, and secondly the inferior gluteal nerve (L5 S1,2) is the nerve supply to gluteus maximus. This very large muscle, which forms the rounded buttock, is the great extensor of the hip joint, acting particularly when rising from a sitting position or climbing up stairs. It is little used in normal walking and, though active in lateral rotation, it has no functional significance in keeping the pelvis correctly balanced during walking.

A haemophiliac develops an expanding haematoma in his psoas muscle, causing pressures on structures deep to the inguinal ligament. On examination, you might expect to find:-

A. loss of sensation in the region of his little toe
B. weakness of dorsiflexion of the foot
C. loss of sensation over the upper lateral side of his thigh
D. weakness in adductor magnus
E. a diminished cremasteric reflex.

Answers overleaf

LL3 Answers

A. & B. FALSE   The region of the little toe on the dorsum of the foot is supplied by the S1 dermatome via the sural nerve. The sural nerve is a cutaneous branch of the tibial division of the sciatic nerve, usually arising in the region of the popliteal fossa. Occasionally, however, a communicating branch is received from the common peroneal branch of the sciatic. The sciatic nerve and its branches leave the pelvis through the greater sciatic foramen, commonly just inferior to piriformis muscle. The muscular branches from the common peroneal include both the deep and superficial peroneal nerves. The anterior compartment muscles which dorsiflex the foot are supplied by the deep peroneal branch, whilst the evertors receive branches from the superficial peroneal nerve.

C. TRUE   The upper lateral skin of the thigh is supplied by the L2, 3, dermatomes via the lateral cutaneous nerve of the thigh. This nerve often forms in the psoas muscle and, emerging from its lateral border, it crosses the posterior pelvic wall towards the anterior superior iliac spine. Here it curves medially to enter the thigh deep to the inguinal ligament, just inferior to the anterior superior iliac spine. Occasionally this nerve pierces the inguinal ligament and severe flexion and extension movements, such as in professional cycling, may result in pain and anaesthesia over the upper thigh (meralgia paraesthetica).

D. FALSE   Adductor magnus commonly is supplied by both the sciatic and obturator nerves. It could be argued that an expanding mass in the psoas muscle might have affected the roots of origin of the obturator, viz, L2, 3, 4 but clinically it is usually the quadriceps which shows weakness in this type of case.

E. TRUE   Stroking the upper medial side of the thigh evokes a reflex contraction of the cremaster muscle, pulling the testis up towards the superficial ring. It is usually more active in children. Its precise value to man is still uncertain, though temperature regulation is often suggested. It is innervated by L1, 2 nerve roots via the femoral and genital branches of the genito-femoral nerve. The genito-femoral nerve is formed deep in psoas muscle, and its femoral branch usually descends on the lateral side of the external iliac artery before passing deep to the inguinal ligament, inside the femoral sheath but lateral to the artery.

In the mid-thigh region the:-

A. floor of the adductor canal is adductor magnus
B. roof of the adductor canal laterally is the vastus medialis
C. femoral artery is medial to its vein and lateral to sartorius muscle
D. iliotibial tract is non-existent
E. gracilis muscle is often supplied by the femoral nerve.

Answers overleaf

A. & B. FALSE & TRUE   The adductor canal or subsartorial canal of Hunter is found medially in the middle third of the thigh. It commences at the apex of the femoral triangle and finishes below at the hiatus in adductor magnus. Its floor is adductor longus and the roof medially is sartorius whilst laterally is situated vastus medialis.

C. TRUE   The contents of this cleft are the femoral artery and vein with the terminal cutaneous branch of the femoral nerve, the saphenous nerve. The nerve to vastus medialis and a small terminal branch of the obturator nerve may also be found. The nerves are normally anterior, the artery medial and the vein situated laterally.

D. FALSE   This noticeable thickening of the fascia lata is easily found during dissection from its superior limits by the tensor fascia lata and gluteus maximus muscles to its insertion in the lateral condyle of the tibia. As it attaches anterior to the axis of the knee joint it assists in keeping the knee extended when the foot is off the ground.

E. FALSE   Gracilis is innervated by the obturator nerve and is in the adductor group though its insertion into the upper shaft of the tibia makes it a weak flexor of the knee joint.

At the ankle joint the:-

A. long saphenous vein is normally situated just posterior to the medial malleolus

B. tibial nerve lies superficial to the flexor retinaculum

C. tendon of peroneus brevis is in direct contact with the fibula

D. extensor hallucis longus is a posterior relation of the dorsalis pedis artery

E. flexor hallucis longus is medial to the flexor digitorum longus.

Answers overleaf

LL5 Answers

A. FALSE   The medial marginal vein of the foot drains the dorsal venous arch into the long saphenous vein. At the ankle it lies 2 – 3 cm anterior to the medial malleolus. It is at this very constant site that 'cut-downs' are usually performed.

B. FALSE   Nearly all structures except the sural and saphenous nerves and veins lie deep to their respective retinacula. Deep to the flexor retinaculum just posterior to the medial malleolus lie, from medial to lateral, tibialis posterior, flexor digitorum longus, posterior tibial artery and veins, tibial nerve and flexor hallucis longus.

C. TRUE   Peroneus brevis and longus both originate from the lateral aspect of the fibula, longus from the upper two thirds, brevis the lower half. Therefore at the ankle the brevis tendon lies deep to longus in direct contact with the bone. Both are involved in eversion. In inversion injuries the insertion of brevis, the base of the fifth metatarsal, is often avulsed.

D. FALSE   The converse is true and it is not until half way down the dorsum of the foot that dorsalis pedis artery may be palpated between extensor hallucis longus and extensor digitorum longus.

E. FALSE   An odd situation but flexor hallucis longus arises from the lateral side of the leg on the posterior aspect of the fibula. It passes deep to the flexor retinaculum and grooves the posterior surface of the talus, before passing forwards hooked under the sustentaculum tali. It crosses deep to the synovial sheath of flexor digitorum longus in the sole of the foot. It is a particularly important muscle in maintaining the medial longitudinal arch. The explanation for this arrangement is that primitively the flexor hallucis sent slips to all five digits but as one climbs the primate tree the muscle begins to lose its lateral tendons and in man normally limits itself to the big toe alone.

A deep intramuscular injection is given into the lower medial quadrant of the buttock and the sciatic nerve is very severely damaged. Conducting your examination you would regrettably expect to find that:-

A. there was severe weakness of adduction
B. flexion of the knee was no longer functional
C. sensation below the knee was completely absent
D. inversion and eversion of the ankle were no longer possible
E. your patient had a marked foot drop.

Answers overleaf

LL6 Answers

A. FALSE   It is true that adductor magnus is supplied by the sciatic nerve but it is also well supplied by the obturator nerve L 2,3,4. The sciatic nerve innervates only the hamstring portion of adductor magnus which originates from the ischial tuberosity and so most of the muscle bulk would be still innervated. Do not forget that adductor longus, adductor brevis and pectineus would be untouched by this injury.

B. TRUE   The major knee flexors are the hamstring muscles—biceps femoris, short and long heads, semimembranosus, and semitendinosus. All of these are sciatic nerve-innervated. The gracilis and sartorius, though assisting in flexion of the knee, would be unlikely to have much effect on their own.

C. FALSE   Though most of the cutaneous supply below the knee is indeed from branches of the sciatic such as the lateral and medial sural, lateral and medial plantar nerves, deep and superficial peroneal nerves, there is one notable exception—the saphenous nerve. This is the cutaneous distal branch of the femoral nerve usually containing L4 fibres. It becomes superficial at the knee and supplies the skin of the medial side of the shin towards the medial malleolus and big toe. (See LL3).

D. TRUE   Inversion is carried out by the tibialis anterior in conjunction with tibialis posterior, extensor hallucis longus and part of extensor digitorum longus. The extensor compartment is supplied by the deep peroneal nerve, a branch of the common peroneal, and the tibialis posterior is innervated via the tibial branch of the sciatic. Eversion is by the peroneal muscles which are supplied by the superficial peroneal nerve.

E. TRUE   Foot drop is caused by loss of dorsiflexion and eversion and damage to the common peroneal branch of the sciatic causes this condition. (See D).

An old lady presents in casualty with a shortened and laterally rotated leg, the classical findings in a case of a subcapital fracture of the neck of the femur. You are concerned that this injury may result in avascular necrosis. All these facts can be explained because the:-

A. ligament of the head supplies about 40% of the blood in the adult
B. major supply of blood is by the medial circumflex artery along the neck deep to the synovial membrane
C. gluteus medius and minimus have rotated the distal fragment laterally
D. piriformis, obturator internus, gamelli, and quadratus femoris have rotated the distal fragment laterally
E. angle between the neck and shaft is about 130° in the adult.

The stability of the normal knee joint is maintained by the:-

A. horizontal inferior fibres of vastus medialis
B. largest sesamoid bone
C. menisci which are very vascular
D. popliteus muscle which 'locks' home the extended knee .
E. fibular collateral ligament which is superficial to the tendon of biceps femoris.

Answers overleaf

LL7 Answers

A. & B. FALSE and TRUE   In the child the femoral epiphysis is supplied by the ligament of the head carrying small branches of the obturator and medial circumflex arteries. When the epiphyseal cartilage matures there is anastomosis between this source and the major supply from the medial circumflex artery. In the adult less than 10% of the supply is from the ligament of the head and so interruption of the vessels deep to the synovial membrane along the neck will cause avascular necrosis.

C. FALSE   Gluteus medius and minimus are abductors, it is maximus which rotates laterally.

D. TRUE   All these muscles and gluteus maximus cause the lateral rotation.

E. TRUE   In the child this angle is increased to about 160°. During fractures of the neck the strong thigh muscles such as quadriceps and hamstrings cause shortening and after healing a decrease in this angle may cause a coxa vara deformity.

LL8 Answers

A. TRUE   These fibres which insert into the patella horizontally actively prevent lateral dislocation of the patella. The height and shape of the lateral condyle also assist.

B. TRUE   The patella is the largest sesamoid bone. Like a seed (Arabic), the sesamoid bones develop in tendons; in the case of the patella ossification takes place around 3 – 4 years of age from several centres as is shown by the occurrence of bipartite patellae. There is much argument as to the usefulness of the patella. It is generally thought to assist full extension and hinder extension from the flexed position.

C. FALSE   Only the lateral margins in contact with the capsule are vascular, in general the menisci are avascular and hence heal poorly following a tear.

D. FALSE   It is the muscle which unlocks the fully extended knee at the commencement of flexion. It does this by rotating the femur laterally on the tibia, if the tibia is fixed as in standing.

E. FALSE   The cord-like fibular collateral ligament extends from the lateral epicondyle to the head of the fibula. Deep to it lies the tendon of popliteus but it is crossed by the biceps femoris tendon. Sometimes there is a bursa between biceps and the ligament (see also LL 1).

84

You are invited to demonstrate to a group of blind physiotherapists the surface markings of the lower limb. Landmarks you suggest would include the:-

A. saphenous opening which lies six finger breadths below and lateral to the symphysis pubis
B. tendon of adductor magnus which is easily palpated in the crutch with the leg abducted
C. site of the posterior inferior iliac spine which is felt as a dimple
D. common peroneal nerve which can normally be rolled against the head of the fibula
E. abductor hallucis muscle which forms the soft concavity of the instep.

LL10 Questions

Lesions of nerves correctly paired with their consequences include:-

A. L4 damage resulting in an absent ankle jerk
B. L2 damage resulting in weakened hip flexion
C. obturator nerve damage alone resulting in little or no sensory loss
D. tibial nerve damage resulting in an absent ankle jerk and a loss of sensation on the sole of the foot
E. S1 damage resulting in an absent ankle jerk and weakness of eversion.

Answers overleaf

LL9 Answers

   A. FALSE   The saphenous opening or cribriform fascia in the fascia lata lies some 3 – 4 finger breadths (3 – 4 cm) below and lateral to the pubic tubercle.

   B. FALSE   The tendon that is so easily felt is that of adductor longus. It is even visible in thin individuals wearing a bathing costume. Adductor magnus is much more fleshy and has no obvious tendon.

   C. FALSE   The 'dimples of Venus' seen or felt in the upper medial quadrant of the buttock are due to fascial adherence to the posterior superior iliac spines. This is also a useful landmark for the level of the 2nd sacral vertebra, the middle of the sacro-iliac joint and the termination of the thecal sac.

   D. FALSE   The common peroneal nerve winds around the neck of the fibula where it may be easily felt.

   E. TRUE

LL10 Answers

   A. FALSE   L4 is the spinal nerve involved in the knee jerk.

   B. TRUE   Damage to L2 affects psoas and iliacus whose combined tendon inserting into the lesser trochanter is a powerful flexor of the hip. Also affected is the femoral nerve (L2,3,4) which supplies rectus femoris, pectineus and sartorius.

   C. TRUE   Remember that all cutaneous sensory supply involves much overlapping between nerves.

   D. TRUE

   E. TRUE   Damage to S1 also involves a loss of sensation just posterior to the lateral malleolus as well as causing problems with plantar flexion.

7. NEUROLOGY

The spinal cord:-

A. in the fetus usually ends at the level of the second lumbar vertebra
B. receives its total arterial blood supply from the vertebral artery or its branches
C. is held in place by the denticulate ligaments of the arachnoid mater
D. has a central canal containing cerebrospinal fluid
E. is surrounded by three meningeal layers and the epidural space which contains many thin walled veins.

Answers overleaf

NR1 Answers

A. FALSE The fetal spinal cord is outgrown by the vertebral column. In the early fetus the cord terminates in the coccygeal region but as the bony column outgrows the cord, by term, the fetal cord usually terminates at L3—L4. This process continues so the adult's cord terminates usually opposite L2 or higher. Flexing of the vertebral column temporarily draws the cord higher so that a lumbar puncture at L3 – L4 in an adult is a relatively unhazardous procedure.

B. FALSE The blood supply of the cord is from three longitudinal arterial channels, one anterior and two posterolaterally. The anterior channel or anterior spinal artery is formed by two branches of the vertebral artery. The posterior spinal arteries are from the vertebral arteries or the posterior inferior cerebellar branches. However, throughout the cord segmental supply by the medullary arteries boost the major longitudinal vessels. These segmental feeders, about twenty in total, are greatest at regions of spinal cord enlargement. The artery of Adamkiewicz or arteria radicularis magna usually arises from a dorsal branch of the posterior intercostal artery at the lower thoracic level. This can be demonstrated by selective arteriography.

C. FALSE It is held in place by the denticulate ligaments, usually 21 on each side but these are formed by the pia and anchor the cord to the arachnoid and dura mater.

D. TRUE The central canal is continuous above with that of the medulla oblongata and thereby with the ventricular system. Below it is sometimes enlarged to form a terminal ventricle, before tapering off into the filum terminale where it ends. In the adult the canal is often obliterated at various levels by proliferation of the lining cells.

E. TRUE The dura, arachnoid and pia mater clothe the spinal cord throughout its length. The epidural or extradural space is between the dura and the bony vertebral canal and contains semifluid fat and numerous thin walled veins of the vertebral venous plexus. It is these veins that may be pierced during a lumbar puncture and cause a false bloody tap.

NR2 Questions

A patient has a right posterior cranial fossa lesion causing pressure on the structures which leave the skull via the jugular foramen. Signs that you would therefore expect to find include:-

A. the tongue deviating to the right
B. an inability to turn the face around towards the left
C. a completely dry mouth and loss of taste over the back of the tongue
D. difficulty in swallowing and speaking
E. problems with hearing.

NR3 Questions

You have a patient with a suspected abnormal CSF who requires lumbar puncture. This proves impossible due to previous spinal surgery and a cisternal tap is considered. Reviewing your anatomy of both the cisterna magna (cerebello-pontine cistern) and the lumbar region you correctly remember that:-

A. the ligamentum nuchae is the cranial extension of the supraspinous ligament alone
B. by mistake you might easily damage the optic chiasma in performing a cisternal puncture
C. the extradural (epidural) space contains numerous small arterial channels
D. in both procedures you must pierce the ligamenta flava
E. the spinal nerve roots in the epidural space are sheathed in dura.

Answers overleaf

NR2 Answers

A. FALSE   Although one of the cranial nerves originating in the medulla is the hypoglossal nerve (XII), it does not leave via the jugular foramen but has its own canal in the occipital bone. The side of the deviation is correct—towards the side of the lesion.

B. TRUE   This is of course the action of sternomastoid muscle on the right side. This muscle is supplied by the spinal root of the accessory nerve, which in company with the vagus and glossopharyngeal leaves the skull through the jugular foramen.

C. FALSE   Rather unfair as you correctly worked out that the glossopharyngeal nerve carries the secretomotor fibres to the parotid (H&N2). However there are six main salivary glands and the loss of one has little effect on the dryness of the mouth. The back of the tongue is also supplied by the glossopharyngeal and even some fibres from the vagus in the region of the valleculae.

D. TRUE   The classical 'bulbar palsy' is due to lesions affecting the vagus and glossopharyngeal which supply the larynx and pharynx respectively.

E. FALSE   You should have listened to your teacher!

NR3 Answers

A. FALSE   The ligamentum nuchae is the cervical extension of both the supra- and interspinous ligaments.

B. FALSE   Only if you had first of all pithed your patient by piercing the medulla and pons. One of the most dangerous aspects of cisternal puncture, especially in children, is the depth of penetration. An over-enthusiastic careless puncture may cause medullary injury resulting in cessation of breathing.

C. FALSE   The extra- or epidural space lies between the spinal dura mater and the periosteum of the vertebral canal. It contains loose fat, areolar tissue and a complex plexus of veins—the internal vertebral venous plexus. It also contains the spinal nerve roots as they cross the space and leave the vertebral canal through each intervertebral foramen.

D. FALSE   Firstly in the upper cervical region there is no ligamentum flavum—it has become the posterior atlanto-occipital membrane; and secondly in the lumbar region the two ligamenta flava lie either side of the midline joining lamina to lamina. If your lumbar puncture is truly midline it will pass between the two ligaments.

E. TRUE

Your patient has a thrombosis of his posterior inferior cerebellar artery and has a classical neurological deficit. You expect to find his problems would include:-

A. difficulty in hearing
B. loss of pain and temperature of the contralateral side to the lesion
C. loss of the sense of smell (anosmia)
D. loss of sight
E. lack of control of the tongue muscles.

NR5 Questions

Fibres passing along the inferior cerebellar peduncle include:-

A. the posterior spino-cerebellar tracts
B. those from the dentate nucleus going to the thalamus
C. those from the dentate nucleus to the cerebral cortex
D. the vestibulo-cerebellar tracts
E. the ponto-cerebellar tracts.

Answers overleaf

NR4 Answers

A. & B. TRUE A posterior inferior cerebellar artery (PICA) thrombosis leads to a 'lateral medullary syndrome'. Structures involved include nuclei ambiguus and solitarius, vestibular and cochlear nuclei, spinal nucleus and the tract of V, spinocerebellar and lateral spinothalmic tracts. Clinically this syndrome is characterised by signs of cranial nerve involvement (V-X), including of course hearing (VIII). The spinothalamic involvement explains the loss of pain and temperature sensitivity. PICA is a very tortuous artery, usually the largest branch of the vertebral and particularly well seen on a lateral vertebral arteriogram where radiologists use it as a marker in posterior fossa lesions since it outlines the anatomy of the brain stem, fourth ventricle and base of the cerebellum.

C. & D. FALSE The cranial nerves more rostally are unaffected.

E. FALSE The area supplied by the PICA in the medulla oblongata lies dorsal to the olivary nucleus and lateral to the hypoglossal nucleus and emerging nerve roots.

NR5 Answers

A. TRUE Tracts in the inferior cerebellar peduncle are passing in both directions but most of those entering have originated in the spinal cord and medulla. These include tracts from the olive, vestibular nucleus, reticular formation and the posterior spinocerebellar columns. These spinocerebellar fibres carry proprioceptive information from the hind limbs and lower trunk. Tracts leaving via this peduncle include those to the olive, vestibular nucleus and reticular formation.

B. & C. FALSE Most fibres in the superior peduncle are leaving the cerebellum and the majority take their cells of origin in the dentate nucleus. Clinically an injury to this nucleus or the superior penduncle itself is a great disability.

D. TRUE See A.

E. FALSE The middle cerebellar penduncle, although physically the largest of the three penduncles, has little variety in its fibres. It is composed almost entirely of second order neurons of the corticopontocerebellar pathway, i.e. fibres relayed from the cortex to the cerebellum via the pontine nuclei.

Your patient has developed a cerebello-pontine angle tumour. It would be likely that his signs and symptoms included:-

A. tinnitus followed later by a progressive deafness
B. vertigo and later ipsilateral ataxia of gait
C. blindness in one eye
D. an absence of corneal reflex
E. twitching of zygomaticus major muscle.

Answers overleaf

NR6 Answers

A. & B. TRUE   The most common, but not only, cause of tumour in this site is an acoustic neuroma. The tumour usually arises on the vestibular division of the VIIIth cranial nerve but the earliest symptoms are auditory. Often a high pitched ringing noise (tinnitus) is followed by progressive deafness. Vertigo due to vestibular damage is rare early in the disease, but later, when the tumour distorts the brainstem and cerebellum, attacks of vertigo, ataxia of gait or of the upper limbs and a mild spastic paraparesis occurs. The ataxia is usually on the limbs of the same side as the lesion.

C. FALSE   The cranial nerves involved in the cerebello-pontine angle are obviously VII and VIII followed by V which is lifted up by the tumour. Occasionally at a later stage VI and IX may be involved.

D. TRUE   This is a fairly consistent early sign due to V being lifted up. It seems that the corneal afferent fibres are particularly sensitive to this distortion. Later it may cause numbness of the face and even weakness in the muscles of mastication.

E. TRUE   Zygomaticus major is a muscle of facial expression and supplied by VII. Twitching of the facial muscles gives rise to a hemifacial spasm. Clinically VII nerve involvement makes the diagnosis of an acoustic neuroma a less likely cause of the tumour.

94

A tumour situated in the rhomboidal floor of the fourth ventricle might well cause some clinical signs. The lesions produced may include:-

A. an inability to whistle
B. an eye which cannot adduct
C. a tongue which deviates on being protruded
D. problems with gastric emptying
E. a drooped upper eyelid (ptosis).

Answers overleaf

NR7 Answers

A. & B. TRUE and FALSE The floor of the fourth ventricle is rhomboidal in shape and is formed by the posterior surface of the pons and the open cranial part of the medulla. It is lined by ependyma and is divided into symmetrical halves by a median sulcus. In its superior part there is an elongated swelling, the facial colliculus, which is due to the ascending facial nerve which winds around the abducent nucleus. A lesion here would therefore produce a facial nerve palsy with inability to whistle, and a lateral rectus palsy causing inability to abduct the eye.

C. TRUE In the inferior part of the floor near the midline is a small triangular swelling, the hypoglossal triangle, deep to which lies the hypoglossal nucleus. The tract of the XII cranial nerve then leaves the medulla between the olive and the pyramid before leaving the skull through the anterior condylar fossa. It is distributed to intrinsic and extrinsic tongue muscles.

D. TRUE Lying also in the inferior part of the floor is the vagal triangle which overlies the dorsal nucleus of the vagus nerve. From this nucleus arise the parasympathetic fibres which travel to the pulmonary, cardiac, oesophageal, gastric and intestinal plexuses. The small ganglia are usually found close to the viscera concerned. The gastric branches are secretomotor to the gastric glands and motor to the muscle coats of the stomach, and as a result of interference with this latter function damage to the vagal nerve converts the stomach into a flaccid bag that empties slowly.

E. FALSE A drooped eyelid may be caused either by sympathetic or third cranial nerve problems. The nucleus of the IIIrd nerve lies in the mid-brain at the level of the superior colliculus and the sympathetic supply to the eyelid is from T1 via the superior cervical ganglia.

In a patient with an expanding pituitary tumour the problems he might develop would include:-

A. an increase in the length of his mandible
B. binasal quadrantic hemianopia
C. erosion of the maxillary sinuses
D. erosion of the posterior clinoid processes
E. rupture of the diaphragma sellae.

NR9 Questions

Horner's Syndrome consists of various physical signs which include a small pupil which reacts normally but over a limited range; drooping of the eyelid (ptosis); a bloodshot conjunctiva, due to loss of vasoconstrictor tone; lack of sweating over the forehead; a sunken eye (enophthalmos), and in congenital cases a paler pigmentation in the iris. Likely causes of such a syndrome are a:-

A. cervical rib
B. T1 cervical cord lesion
C. lateral brain stem lesion
D. cavernous sinus lesion
E. superior cervical ganglion transection.

Answers overleaf

97

NR8 Answers

A. TRUE   Difficulty in eating due to changes in the proportions of the bones involved is a classical presentation of an acidophil adenoma. Acromegaly is characterised by overgrowth of the frontal sinuses, jaw and distal phalanges.

B. FALSE   Tumours of the pituitary often cause blindness due to its site just postero-inferior to the optic chiasma. However the vision problem is caused by pressure on the inferior aspect of the chiasma which leads to atrophy of the nerve fibres from the lower nasal quadrants of the retina. The result is that the patient loses the upper temporal quadrants of his field of vision while leaving his nasal fields untouched—bitemporal quadrantic hemianopia.

C: FALSE   The sphenoidal air sinus is the inferior relation of the pituitary fossa.

D. & E. TRUE   The pituitary or hypophyseal gland lies in sella turcica or hypophyseal fossa whose boundaries include the anterior and posterior clinoid processes of bone. Stretched across the roof of this fossa and attached to the bone is a dural layer—the diaphragma sellae.

NR9 Answers

A. & B. TRUE   Any interruption of either T1, cord or root, will produce a Horner's syndrome. In the cord central lesions may cause a bilateral Horner's and in the roots involvement of the lower trunk of the brachial plexus by tumour (See TH 9), a cervical rib, or injury (Klumpke's paralysis) will cause a unilateral Horner's.

C. TRUE   The first order neuron lies adjacent to the spino-thalamic tracts in the brain stem and presenting symptoms will often include loss of pain and temperature on the other side of the body.

D. TRUE   The sympathetics travel around the internal carotid artery as it passes through the cavernous sinus.
Thrombosis of the artery or even migraine spasms in this region may produce the condition.

E. TRUE

8. HISTOLOGY

HISTO1 Questions

The cells of the APUD system:-

A. have high levels of both rough endoplasmic reticulum and free ribosomes
B. include the C cells in the thyroid
C. can take up amine precursors
D. contain an amino acid carboxylase
E. secrete gastrin, which is also found in the cerebral cortex.

HISTO2 Questions

When looking down the microscope at normal tissue stained with haemotoxylin and eosin one would see that:-

A. in the parotid gland there are only rare fat cells
B. in the submandibular gland most alveoli are mucus secreting
C. in the sublingual gland most alveoli are mucus secreting
D. in both the pancreas and parotid glands there are serous acini with pyramidal-shaped cells
E. in the lacrimal gland the acinar lumina are conspicuous.

Answers overleaf

99

HISTO1 Answers

A. FALSE   In the APUD cell system we find low levels of rough endoplasmic reticulum, but high levels of both smooth endoplasmic reticulum and free ribosomes. These morphological characteristics are not truly specific to the APUD system cells, but are seen in most protein-secreting cells.

B. TRUE   The C cells secrete calcitonin and in the bird it has been shown that the ultimobranchial gland containing these cells is of neural crest origin. It is likely that a similar situation exists in man.

C. & D. TRUE and FALSE   APUD stands for (A) Contains a fluorogenic *a*mine such as 5HT, or can at least secondarily take it up. (PU) Can take up amine precursors, e.g. DOPA, i.e. *p*recursor *u*ptake (D) contains an amino acid *d*ecarboxylase.

E. TRUE   Many of the APUD peptides originally found in the gut have now been isolated from the brain. Such peptides include—substance P, somatostatin, gastrin and VIP.

HISTO2 Answers

A. FALSE   One of the most difficult groups of tissues to distinguish are the secreting glands. The parotid gland contains only serous acini with pyramidal-shaped cells and normally contains numerous fat cells

B. & C. FALSE and TRUE   The sudmandibular gland contains mostly serous with just a few mucous alveoli. In comparison, the parotid is all serous and the sublinguinal gland has usually slightly more mucous than serous alveoli. Mixed alveoli are commonly seen in both submandibular and sublingual glands, the serous cells capping the mucous alveoli forming the so-called 'demilunes' or half-moons.

D. & E. TRUE   It may be very difficult to distinguish the parotid from the pancreas or lacrimal gland, both of which have only serous acini. The cells of the lacrimal gland are, however, not pyramidal but columnar cells with basal nuclei. The acinar lumina of the parotid are minute, whereas those of the lacrimal gland are conspicuous; neither contain centroacinar cells, which are diagnostic of the pancreas. Another obvious distinguishing feature of the pancreas is the pale-staining areas of the islets of Langerhans.

The myelin sheath surrounding an axon:-

A. is formed in the central nervous system by an astrocyte
B. is proportional in thickness to the axon diameter
C. has no nodes of Ranvier in the central nervous system (CNS).
D. is usually surrounded by collagen fibres in the central nervous system
E. contains fissures or clefts in both peripheral and central nervous systems.

Answers overleaf

HISTO3 Answers

A. The myelin sheath in CNS fibres is formed by processes from oligodendrocytes. Though the exact mechanism is in dispute it is generally believed that attenuated processes of the oligodendrocyte wrap themselves around the axon. A single cell may be responsible for the myelin sheath in many different axons.

B. TRUE   A small diameter axon may have only a few myelin layers or lamellae whereas a large peripheral nerve fibre may be sheathed by sixty or more lamellae. These concentric layers of myelin, as seen by electron microscopy with stainings, can be distinguished into minor and major dense lines. A lamella is from one major dense line to the next.

C. & D.   FALSE   In the CNS there is but little collagen, and that is found around large blood vessels and not in the extracellular fluid, as is commonly seen in the peripheral nerve. In the peripheral nerve two adjoining Schwann cells on the same axon are separated by a node of Ranvier where they can be seen to interdigitate. The Schwann cells' formation of the myelin sheath is believed to act as an insulator causing saltatory conduction of the impulse from node to node. In the C.N.S., though often more difficult to find, a similar arrangement exists whereby two oligodendrocyte processes lie either side of a node of Ranvier.

E.   TRUE   In both CNS and peripheral nerves there are oblique fissures in the myelin sheath called Schmidt-Lantermann clefts. Here the lamellae are not so compacted and Schwann cell cytoplasm lies in the clefts.

Presented with a tissue containing non-keratinized stratified squamous epithelium and skeletal muscle fibres, you would deduce that it could have been prepared from the:-

A. vagina
B. lower lip
C. tongue
D. upper third of the oesophagus
E. skin of the scalp.

Answers overleaf

HISTO4 Answers

A. FALSE   Although the vaginal epithelum is non-keratinized stratified squamous, its muscle fibres are smooth, not skeletal. Other features often seen on a vaginal section include a prominent venous plexus, and loose connective tissue which is rich in lymphocytes and the occasional lymph nodule. Naturally the vaginal epithelium undergoes cyclic changes during the menstrual cycle.

B. C. & D.   TRUE   The epithelium which lines the digestive tract from lips as far as the oesophagus is non-keratinized stratified squamous epithelum. At the junction with the stomach there is a sharp transition to columnar epithelium. The lip can be distinguished by the numerous arteries, conspicuous collagenous fibres and the mucous, labial glands. Peculiar to the tongue are the numerous papillae: filiform, fungiform and vallate, as well as both mucous and serous glands lying in a bed of fibro-fatty connective tissue. In the case of the oesophagus the external muscle layer is made up entirely of skeletal muscle in the upper third; of skeletal and smooth muscle fibres in the middle third; and of purely smooth muscle in the lower third. Although typically described as an inner circular and outer longitudinal muscle layer, many of the bundles are arranged obliquely or in a spiral fashion. Between the two muscle layers one may find numerous small ganglia associated with the myenteric nerve plexus (Auerbach).

E. FALSE   The skin of the scalp is keratinized stratified squamous epithelium. The epidermal layer of skin varies in thickness from one site to another, the palms and soles for instance being the thickest. In these regions four layers of the epidermis can be easily defined, viz. strata Malpighii, granulosum, lucidum and corneum.

Stained histological sections of normal bowel tissue, viewed with the light microscope, reveal that:-

A. there are numerous sinuses in the wall of the gall bladder
B. the jejunum often contains Peyer's patches
C. the ileum contains numerous glands in the sub-mucosa
D. the body of the stomach has many chief and parietal cells
E. the ileum has three distinct muscle layers.

Answers overleaf

HISTO5 Answers

A. TRUE   The salient features of the gall bladder are that it has no true villi, but mucosal folds resembling villi, no goblet cells, except in the neck region, and numerous diverticula or sinuses. It does not have a submucosa, and a small muscle layer lies adjacent to the lamina propria.

B. FALSE   Peyer's patches are aggregations of lymphoid tissue found in the ileum, not the jejunum. However, lymphoid tissue in the form of solitary lymph nodules is seen in the duodenum and jejunum.

C. FALSE   The ileum contains no glands in the submucosa. These Brunner's glands are most prominent in the duodenum, where they are diagnostic.

D. TRUE   This is also true of the fundus of the stomach, whereas the pylorus has fewer of these cells.

E. FALSE   The ileum has only two muscle layers, an inner circular and an outer longitudinal layer. It is in the stomach that a third oblique layer may be found.

You are shown some stained tissue preparations the features of which include a true ciliated border and smooth muscle fibres. These sections are therefore taken from the:-

A. epididymis
B. ampulla of the oviduct
C. small respiratory bronchioles
D. vas deferens
E. tongue.

Answers overleaf

HISTO6 Answers

A. FALSE Both the epididymis and vas have pseudostratified columnar cells with a border of stereocilia. These are non-motile processes of the columnar cells projecting into the lumen. Although called cilia, electron microscopy has now shown that they lack the fine structural characteristics seen in all cilia and are really very long microvilli. The ultrastructure of all cilia in both plant and animal kingdoms consists of two central filaments surrounded by nine paired ones. The function of the stereocilia is not well established but the epididymal epithelium is absorptive and it is assumed that these stereocilia promote this function by increasing the cell surface area.

B. TRUE The epithelium is of the simple columnar variety and usually consists of two cell types. One of these, especially numerous on the fimbriae and in the ampulla, has cilia that beat towards the uterus. The other cell type is devoid of cilia and thought to be secretory. This epithelium undergoes cyclic changes and the relative proportions of ciliated to non-ciliated is under endocrine control. Monkey studies have shown that, in the late luteal phase of the cycle, the fimbrial epithelium becomes devoid of cilia. The oviduct wall consists of mucosa, a smooth muscle layer, and an external serous coat.

C. FALSE Normal respiratory epithelium such as seen in the bronchus and bronchioles consists of ciliated pseudostratified columnar epithelium. In the small bronchioles the epithelium is simple columnar ciliated and the lamina propria is replaced by a smooth muscle layer which encircles the bronchiole. In man, cartilage and glands are often present until the bronchiole decreases in size to about 0.5 mm in diameter. A respiratory bronchiole is a branch of the terminal bronchiole. The epithelium is from low columnar to low cuboidal and cilia are only present in the larger respiratory bronchioles. The thin supporting wall of the respiratory bronchiole consists of collagenous and elastic fibres with some smooth muscle.

D. FALSE (see A)

E. FALSE This is wrong on both counts. The epithelium of the tongue is stratified squamous and non-ciliated. Although the papillae might be confused with cilia they are easily distinguished even at the light microscope level. The filiform papillae are made up of a thin core of vascularised connective tissue covered by a cornified stratified squamous epithelium. The muscle fibres of the tongue are striated and consist of interwoven bundles of fibres in all three directions: longitudinal, transverse and vertical.

It is demonstrable in sections of muscle tissue stained with haematoxylin and eosin (H & E) that:-

A. smooth muscle has uniform nuclei and a homogenous cytoplasm
B. cross striations are prominent in smooth muscle
C. the nuclei seen in skeletal muscle are fusiform
D. cardiac muscle has branching fibres and peripheral nuclei
E. cardiac and skeletal muscle both have cross striations.

Answers overleaf

HISTO7 Answers

A. & B. TRUE and FALSE   When comparing stained sections of skeletal, cardiac and smooth muscle it is quite easy to distinguish smooth muscle from either of the others by its homogenous cytoplasm. The nuclei of smooth muscle are centrally placed, fusiform in shape and are normally fairly uniform in size.

C. FALSE   Skeletal muscle has small peripheral nuclei, non-branching fibres and its most prominent staining feature is cross striations. The A and I bands and the Z lines can be seen using this stain. The reduction of the distance between Z lines denotes the degree of contraction.

D. & E. FALSE and TRUE   Cardiac muscle has centrally placed nuclei, obvious branching fibres and only faint cross striations compared with those seen in skeletal muscle. It also has the unique feature of the intercalated disc which is the junctional site between the fibres. This disc is composed of two important components; the adhesion plate or desmosome between adjacent cells and the nexus or gap junction. These junctions assist in both electrical and mechanical cell-to-cell cohesion thus enabling the myocardium to behave as though it were a syncytium.

Correct associations in histological slides include:-

A. thymus—Hassall's corpuscle
B. portal canal—Glisson's capsule
C. lactating mammary gland—saccular alveoli
D. thyroid gland—squamous lined ducts
E. organ of Corti—perilymphatic space.

Answers overleaf

HISTO8 Answers

A. TRUE   In the medulla of the thymus is found a structure unique to this organ, the Hassall's corpuscle. It is composed of epithelioid cells arranged in layers with a dense hyalinized core, surrounded by flattened cells. These corpuscles tend to increase in both size and number with age.

B. TRUE   At the periphery of the hepatic lobule are the portal canals which contain branches of the hepatic artery, the thin-walled portal vein and a bile duct. Sometimes a small lymph vessel may also be found. These portal canals are surrounded by Glisson's capsule which is composed of dense collagenous fibres.

C. TRUE   In the active lactating stage the alveoli of the breast become saccular and are distended by the secretions of milk.

D. FALSE   There are neither ducts nor lobules in the thyroid gland. The structural units of this gland are the follicles which are filled with clear hyaline colloid. This colloid is in fact a glycoprotein-iodine complex.

E. FALSE   The organ of Corti is within the scala media or cochlear duct and is part of the endolymphatic system. The scala vestibuli and scala tympani are perilymphatic spaces, extending to the inner surfaces of the oval and round windows respectively.

9. EMBRYOLOGY

EMB1 Questions

Structures derived from the paramesonephric duct are the:-

A. round ligament of the uterus
B. Gartner's duct
C. prostatic utricle
D. epoöphoron
E. seminal vesicle.

EMB2 Questions

The second branchial arch derivatives include the:-

A. mandibular nerve
B. posterior belly of digastric muscle
C. greater cornu of the hyoid bone
D. tensor veli palatini
E. stylohyoid ligament.

Answers overleaf

EMB1 Answers

A. FALSE   The round ligament of the uterus is one of the remnants of the gubernaculum, the other being the ovarian ligament.

B. FALSE   Gartner's duct is a remnant of the mesonephros (Wolffian duct), the caudal part of which degenerates slowly and forms this duct which may be traced alongside the female genital tract from the epoöphoron to the hymen.

C. TRUE   The prostatic utricle or little uterus is a 1 cm diverticulum within the urethral crest of the prostatic gland. Onto the lips of the utricle open the pinpoint orifices of the two ejaculatory ducts. Each duct, whose diameter is about the size of the lead in a pencil, is the final common pathway of the seminal vesicle and ampullae of the vas of each side. The prostatic utricle and the appendages of the epididymis and testes are the only remnants of the paramesonephric ducts (Mullerian) in the male.

D. FALSE   Epoöphoron (above the egg basket) is found in the broad ligament and is a remnant in the female of the mesonephros (Wolffian body).

E. FALSE   The seminal vesicles are formed from the mesonephric duct and each in fact is a diverticulum developed from the ampullated end of the ductus deferens. An easy way to remember which duct contributes to male or female genital development is that men are always wolves and hence the most male organs develop from the Wolffian or mesonephric duct!

EMB2 Answers

A. FALSE   The mandibular nerve is associated with the muscles of mastication and these are all of first arch origins. The nerve associated with the second arch is the facial nerve.

B. TRUE   The muscles of the second arch are those of facial expression and include all of those around the eye, nose and mouth used in facial movements but also the posterior belly of digastric, stylohyoid, stapedius and platysma.

C. FALSE   The greater cornu is from the third branchial arch. It is the lesser cornu and body which originate from the second arch.

D. FALSE   Tensor veli palatini is a muscle of mastication and of first arch origin supplied by the trigeminal nerve, mandibular branch.

E. TRUE   The second branchial arch cartilage derivatives include: stapes, styloid process, stylohyoid ligament and the lesser cornu of the hyoid.

114

Neural crest tissue contributes to the:-

A. pharyngeal arches
B. segmental spinal ganglia
C. odontoblasts
D. cutaneous melanoblasts
E. nucleus pulposus.

Answers overleaf

EMB3 Answers

A. B. C. & D. TRUE As the neural groove indents and the neural plate cells migrate to form the neural tube, a series of segmented primordia are left lying dorsolateral to the tube. These cells form all the spinal and most of the cranial sensory ganglia as well as the origins of both sympathetic and parasympathetic ganglia. In the segmental spinal ganglia the crest cells form bipolar neuroblasts whose processes complete the dorsal roots of the spinal nerves. In company with autonomic neuroblasts, some of the neural crest tissue differentiates into the chromaffin cells of the abdominal aorta and the largest mass of these cells forms the adrenal medulla. The Schwann cell of the peripheral nerve is also of neural crest origin. It also forms cutaneous melanoblasts, dental papillae and odontoblasts as well as contributing to the pharyngeal arches, particularly their cartilages. Finally, the neural crest gives rise, in part at least, to the meninges.

E. FALSE The mistake here is to confuse the cells of the neural crest with those of the notochord which lies anterior to the neural tube. It is the notochord which forms the skeleton for the vertebrae and, more specifically, the centrum of the vertebrae. During development the notochord becomes surrounded by a mass of mesenchyme which is later subdivided by intervertebral fissures. After much differential growth the notochordal cells undergo mucoid degeneration and form part of the nucleus pulposus within the annulus fibrosus of the intervertebral disc. As the vertebrae themselves become cartilaginous the centrum ossifies and the notochord regresses as the body of the vertebra is formed.

In the fetal circulation:-

A. the left umbilical vein drains into the ductus venosus
B. the septum secundum grows down as the limbus of the foramen ovale
C. the right ventricular wall is at least as thick as the left ventricular wall
D. at birth the umbilical arteries contract before the umbilical vein
E. the highest oxygen saturation is in the umbilical vein.

Answers overleaf

EMB4 Answers

A. TRUE   The remaining umbilical vein taking blood from the placenta towards the liver and heart is the left one. The blood bypasses the liver to the post-hepatic inferior vena cava via the ductus venosus which, following birth, obliterates, becoming the ligamentum venosum.

B. TRUE   The sickle-shaped septum secundum grows down as the limbus of the foramen ovale. The septum primum lies on its left side, forming a flap-like valve. At birth the functional closure of the foramen ovale is dependent on the onset of respiration. Although this functional closure occurs at birth it is not until the left atrial pressure rises that any remaining shunt ceases and the valve begins to fuse with the limbus. However, even in the adult, though functionally closed, it is possible in some 20% of people to find an anatomical channel still patent.

C. TRUE   At birth, the right ventricle outweighs the left; however, within a month the left is heavier, due to ventricular hypertrophy. By six months the relative left ventricular wall thickness seen in later life has been established. These differences are due to pressure changes within the pulmonary and systemic arteries.

D. TRUE   The arteries contract before the vein or ductus venosus. An appreciable volume of fetal blood is liable to return from the placenta if the cord is not clamped immediately.

E. TRUE   The approximate percentage oxygen saturation figures for various vessels in the fetal circulation include: umbilical vein — 80, post-hepatic inferior vena cava — 70, pulmonary trunk — 50, superior vena cava — 30.

During development of the fetal skull the:-

A. parietal bone forms in membrane
B. interparietal portion of the occipital bone forms in cartilage
C. lesser wing of the sphenoid forms in cartilage
D. tympanic part of the temporal bone forms in cartilage
E. mandible forms in membrane around a cartilaginous core.

Answers overleaf

EMB5 Answers

A. B. & C. TRUE, FALSE and TRUE The primitive fetal skull can be divided into its neurocranial and viscerocranial elements. The vault of the neurocranium develops in membrane, i.e. frontal, parietal and interparietal part of the occipital bone. The cartilaginous neurocranial elements include the nasal and otic capsules and the definitive occipital bone (except the interparietal part); the petromastoid portions of the temporal bone; body, lesser wings and roots of the greater wings of the sphenoid bone; ethmoid and inferior concha.

D. FALSE The viscerocranium can be divided into its cartilaginous elements formed from the pharyngeal arch cartilage, and the facial bones which develop in membrane. The temporal bone is a good example of this division. The squamous and tympanic parts of the temporal bone develop in membrane, its petromastoid parts in neurocranial cartilage and the styloid process is a second pharyngeal arch cartilage derivative.

E. TRUE Meckel's cartilage is a first pharyngeal arch cartilage derivative and forms the core to the primitive lower jaw. The proximal end of this cartilage forms the malleus whereas the distal portion becomes surrounded by and later invaded by the membranous ossification of the mandible.

Six weeks after conception in the human embryo the:-

A. heart will have just started to beat
B. haemopoiesis will be located in the bone marrow
C. external genitalia are distinctive
D. midgut loop herniates
E. neural tube is closed.

Answers overleaf

EMB6 Answers

A. TRUE   At approximately six weeks the cardiac muscle is fully developed and starts beating.

B. FALSE   Haemopoiesis is found at different sites during development, but it is not until about 12 – 14 weeks that the bone marrow is involved. At first certain mesenchyme cells in the yolk sac differentiate into haemocytoblasts. These cells accumulate haemoglobin and enter the large-celled primitive erythrocyte series. The yolk sac haemopoiesis is during the first three months, overlapping with the liver which is involved from one month to birth. The spleen is another site during the mid-trimester and it is not until three months that the bone marrow and lymphoid tissue are involved.

C. FALSE   It is not until about three months that the external genitalia are distinctive. Nowadays this fact is being used in sex determination, by ultrasound after fourteen weeks.

D. TRUE   At about six weeks the midgut loop forms, its apex being continuous with the vitello-intestinal duct. This loop elongates very rapidly at the same time as the primitive liver and kidney are enlarging. As a consequence, the loop and its dorsal mesentery are extruded into the extraembryonic coelom which persists in the umbilical cord. This extrusion is the physiological herniation of the midgut.

E. TRUE   The neural tube closes around the fourth week after conception.

During development of the arteries:-

A. there are two dorsal aortae
B. the aortic sac contributes to the definitive pulmonary trunk
C. the ductus arteriosus is formed from the left sixth aortic arch
D. the right subclavian artery is formed from the right sixth aortic arch
E. the internal carotid artery is formed from the dorsal aorta and third aortic arch.

Answers overleaf

EMB7 Answers

A. TRUE   The aortic arch arteries develop in mesenchyme and connect the two dorsal aortae with the aortic sac. Between the upper thoracic and lower lumbar segments they fuse to form the single descending aorta.

B. TRUE   During the growth of the neck and descent of the heart, the third and fourth arch arteries draw out the aortic sac on each side to form horns which become the brachiocephalic and left common carotid arteries in the fetus. The aortic sac also contributes to the origin of the pulmonary trunk.

C. & D. TRUE and FALSE   The sixth aortic arch arteries are atypical. At first they supply primitive pulmonary plexuses and only later connect up to the dorsal aortae. The ventral parts become the pulmonary arteries. On the right side, connection to the dorsal aorta disappears, but on the left it persists as the ductus arteriosus. As the fifth pair of aortic arch arteries is absent or at best very transient in man, one can easily explain the asymmetrical position of the recurrent laryngeal nerves. On the left the recurrent laryngeal nerve hooks around the ductus arteriosus, not the aorta, as it is a sixth branchial arch nerve. On the right, however, because of the disappearance of the fifth and sixth arch arteries it can hook around the left subclavian artery which is formed mainly from the fourth arch artery.

E. TRUE   Its dorsal portion also has contribution from first and second arches.

A normal girl aged 4 has X-rays of her hands and feet. The centres of ossification that you would expect to see include:-

A. cuboid
B. scaphoid
C. a sesamoid bone in the foot
D. lunate
E. navicular.

Answers overleaf

EMB8 Answers

A. TRUE   The cuboid usually appears at or around birth. Other centres of ossification at about this time include the head of the humerus and the proximal end of the tibia. The distal end of the femur is normally before birth.

B. TRUE   Had this question been about a 4-year-old boy, then the chances are that his scaphoid would not have appeared. Approximately 50% of 4 year old girls have the scaphoid visible. This figure is not reached until tne age of 6 in boys.

C. FALSE   The sesamoid bones in both hands and feet do not appear until about the age of 9 or 10. Girls' sesamoids tend to ossify earlier and the foot sesamoids prior to those in the hand.

D. TRUE   By 4, nearly all young girls have a visible lunate on X-ray. As a rule, only about half the boys X-rayed would have this centre of ossification.

E. TRUE   The navicular bone appears around the age of 2 to 3 years. As a general rule, ladies before gentlemen in both centres of ossification and fusion dates.

II. PHYSIOLOGY

1. RESPIRATORY

The intrapleural pressure:-

A. is always negative (i.e. subatmospheric)
B. increases (i.e. becomes less negative) on deep inspiration
C. increases (i.e. becomes less negative) on performing the Valsalva manoeuvre (forced expiration against a closed glottis)
D. can be measured with a catheter in the oesophagus
E. changes at high altitudes.

In the respiratory system, physiological shunt:-

A. is smaller than the anatomical shunt
B. is not present in the healthy adult
C. affects arterial carbon dioxide more than arterial oxygen tension
D. has the same effect on respiratory gas exchange as does physiological dead space
E. is abolished when the subject breathes pure oxygen.

Answers overleaf

R1 Answers

A. FALSE During strong expiratory efforts, as in coughing or performing Valsalva's manoeuvre (see C) the intrapleural pressure may rise to the atmospheric level and above.

B. As the chest wall moves outward during inspiration the intrapleural pressure falls to become even more negative.

C. TRUE (See A above)

D. TRUE

E. FALSE The mechanical properties of chest wall and lung are independent of the ambient pressure.

R2 Answers

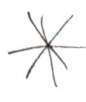

A. FALSE Physiological shunt is the sum of the *anatomical* shunt (blood passing from the right ventricle to the systemic circulation via normal anatomical pathways, e.g. the bronchial vessels, the Thebesian veins, without passing through the pulmonary alveolar capillaries), and the element of pulmonary alveolar capillary blood that has passed through non- or poorly aerated alveoli. Therefore physiological shunt is always at least as great as, or greater than the anatomical shunt.

B. FALSE There is always a normal anatomical shunt, at least, and even in the young healthy adult there is probably some contribution in excess of this through poorly aerated alveoli.

C. FALSE The difference in carbon dioxide tension between arterial and mixed venous blood is a little less than 1 kPa (6 mm Hg), and therefore even a 50% shunt only increases arterial carbon dioxide tension by about 0.5 k Pa (3 m.Hg). A 50% shunt would reduce arterial oxygen tension from 13.5 kPa (100 mm Hg) to below 9 kPa (70 mm Hg).

D. FALSE Physiological dead space results primarily in a failure to remove carbon dioxide from alveolar gas, i.e. a rise in arterial carbon dioxide tension, if ventilation is not increased.

E. FALSE The breathing of pure oxygen cannot eliminate the anatomical right-to-left portion of the physiological shunt (see answer A above).

In the lungs, the physiological dead space is:-

A. synonymous with the term 'physiological shunt'
B. likely to decrease in old age
C. increased by intermittent positive pressure ventilation
D. increased in hypovolaemic shock
E. greater in the erect than in the supine position.

The oxygen content of a sample of blood:-

A. is always greater at a higher oxygen partial pressure than at a lower
B. is always twice as great when the oxygen partial pressure is doubled
C. at a fixed partial pressure of oxygen is lower at lower pH
D. at a fixed partial pressure of oxygen is lower at lower temperature
E. at a fixed partial pressure of oxygen is lower at lower partial pressure of carbon dioxide.

Answers overleaf

R3 Answers

A. FALSE 'Physiological shunt' is the admixture in the peripheral arterial blood that has not been properly oxygenated because it has passed through the pulmonary capillaries of alveoli that are poorly, or not at all, ventilated, or has passed through anatomical shunt pathways. Thus physiological shunt is the opposite ventilation/perfusion imbalance to physiological dead space.

B. FALSE Physiological dead space tends to increase in old age.

C. TRUE The increased external pressure tends to cause collapse of the pulmonary arterioles, especially those near the apices of the lungs where the factor of gravity is strongest; the affected alveoli are still ventilated but their capillary perfusion has ceased, i.e. the alveolar dead space has increased.

D. TRUE The reduced cardiac output results in a reduction of pulmonary arterial pressure with the same results as in C.

E. TRUE See C above for the effect of gravity, which will be greater in the erect position.

R4 Answers

A. TRUE Even when the sigmoid part of the oxygen-dissociation curve has been passed (i.e. at oxygen tensions greater than 13.5 kPa, 100 mm Hg), increasing oxygen tension increases the amount of oxygen dissolved in the water of blood, and hence the total oxygen content.

B. FALSE The relation between oxygen tension and oxygen content is not linear but an S-shaped curve.

C. TRUE This is the Bohr effect.

D. FALSE The converse is true.

E. FALSE The converse is true. Thus, C D & E can be remembered as factors that reduce oxygen content (i.e. increase oxygen availability to tissues) in conditions where the tissue is engaged in metabolic activity and so raising hydrogen ion concentration, raising temperature and raising carbon dioxide concentration.

Adaptations to chronic anoxia at altitudes of about **14 000 feet (4500 m)** include:-

A. a marked increase in ventilation rate (about 30 – 40%)   T
B. an increased sensitivity of the respiratory centre to arterial carbon dioxide tension
C. a well-maintained increase in cardiac output
D. an increased output of erythropoeitin   T
E. an increased concentration of 2,3-diphosphoglycerate (2,3-DPG) T in erythrocytes.

In the pulmonary alveoli the partial pressure of:-

A. oxygen is approximately the same as in the atmosphere
B. nitrogen is approximately the same as in the atmosphere
C. carbon dioxide is within about 1 mm Hg (0.1 kPa) the same as mixed venous blood
D. oxygen is a few millimetres of mercury higher than in the arterial blood in a healthy young adult
E. water vapour depends only upon the temperature.

Answers overleaf

R5 Answers

A. TRUE In this respect, chronic anoxia differs from acute anoxia, which only increases ventilation by about 10%. The mechanism whereby chronic anoxia increases ventilation rate is not clear.

B. TRUE This effect helps to maintain a high rate of ventilation despite the concomitant lowering of the arterial carbon dioxide tension.

C. FALSE By the time adaptation is complete, cardiac output, which is initially raised, has returned to normal.

D. TRUE Hypoxia stimulates an increased output of the hormone, erythropoetin, in the kidneys: erythropoetin in turn stimulates the bone marrow to produce more erythrocytes.

E. TRUE 2,3-DPG has the property of shifting the oxygen dissociation curve of haemoglobin to the right: i.e. the amount of oxygen given up to the tissues at low P_{O_2} is increased.

R6 Answers

A. FALSE The majority of the difference between oxygen partial pressure in atmosphere and alveoli is due to the gaseous exchange of oxygen for carbon dioxide between alveolar gas and pulmonary arterial capillaries.

B. TRUE Nitrogen is an inert gas, and apart from minor effects due to water vapour and to the change in volume produced by the unequal exchange of oxygen and carbon dioxide, the nitrogen partial pressures are the same in the atmosphere and the alveoli.

C. FALSE P_{CO_2} is higher in mixed venous blood than in pulmonary alveoli by 6 mm Hg (about 1 kPa), and this provides the gradient to drive carbon dioxide from the blood into the alveoli. If you got this wrong, you were probably thinking of the fact that alveolar P_{CO_2} is practically the same as *arterial* P_{CO_2}.

D. TRUE There is a small alveolo-arterial oxygen tension gradient due to some right-to-left shunting in poorly ventilated alveoli at the bases of the lungs and to minor anatomical shunts, e.g. in Thebesian and bronchial veins, but in young healthy adults the gradient is 2 or 3 mm only.

E. TRUE The alveolar gas is saturated with water vapour and saturated water vapour pressure is fixed by temperature—e.g. 47 mm Hg (6.5 kPa) at 37°C.

The rate at which a gas diffuses across the pulmonary alveolo-capillary membrane is:-

A. independent of temperature
B. proportional to the solubility of the gas in body fluids
C. proportional to the molecular weight of the gas
D. inversely proportional to the thickness of the membrane
E. dependent on any chemical reactions in which the gas takes part in the blood.

With a subject breathing quietly at rest:-

A. the volume of gas inspired and expired with each breath is called the tidal volume
B. the volume of gas remaining in his lungs after quiet expiration is called the functional residual capacity (FRC)
C. the FRC can be measured by nitrogen wash-out techniques (i.e. breathing pure oxygen)
D. after quiet inspiration, the volume of gas he can breathe in as a result of a maximal inspiratory effort is called the vital capacity
E. expiration requires no muscular effort.

Answers overleaf

R7 Answers

A. FALSE   The velocity of molecules in a gas is proportional to the temperature and so a higher temperature facilitates diffusion.

B. TRUE   Carbon dioxide diffuses much more rapidly than oxygen because it is much more soluble.

C. FALSE   The rate of diffusion of a gas is *inversely* proportional to the square root of its molecular weight.

D. TRUE

E. TRUE   As the gas takes part in the chemical reaction, its concentration (partial pressure) in the blood is kept low and this facilitates diffusion across the alveolo-capillary membrane.

R8 Answers

A. TRUE

B. TRUE

C. TRUE   A consequence of breathing in pure oxygen is that the nitrogen in the lungs is gradually 'washed out'. The volume of the FRC can be worked out from the rate at which the proportion of nitrogen in the expired gas falls.

D. FALSE   The volume described is the *inspiratory reserve volume*. The *vital capacity* is the volume expired as a result of a maximal expiratory effort after a maximal inspiratory effort.

E. TRUE   The factors producing the return of the lung to its normal size are its inherent elasticity, the surface tension of its moist alveoli, and the elasticity of the chest wall.

Using the Fick principle, data required for an accurate measurement of cardiac output include oxygen:-

A. consumption
B. content of blood from brachial artery
C. content of blood from coronary sinus
D. content of blood from pulmonary artery
E. content of blood from femoral vein.

Answers overleaf

R9 Answers

A. TRUE ⎫
B. TRUE ⎪ The Fick principle states that the cardiac output
C. FALSE ⎬ can be derived from the arteriovenous difference
D. TRUE ⎪ in concentration of any substance divided into
E. FALSE ⎭ the rate at which that substance is added to, or

removed from, the circulation. In mathematical
terms, for oxygen:

$$\text{Oxygen (ml/min) consumed} = \left\{ \begin{array}{c} \text{arterial} \\ \text{oxygen ml/l} \\ \text{content} \end{array} - \begin{array}{c} \text{venous} \\ \text{oxygen ml/l} \\ \text{content} \end{array} \right\} \times \begin{array}{c} \text{cardiac} \\ \text{output} \end{array} \text{ml/min}$$

$$\begin{array}{c} \text{cardiac} \\ \text{output} \end{array} = \frac{\text{oxygen consumption}}{\text{arterial—venous oxygen content}}$$

Thus A is true and so is B since arterial oxygen content does not appreciably differ between one artery and any other. However, for venous oxygen content the correct sample to obtain is mixed venous blood returned from all over the body, immediately before it is exposed to the pulmonary alveolar oxygenation process. Thus D is true, but because of variations in the extent of oxygen extraction from individual regions of the body such as the lower limb or the myocardium, C & E are false; such samples may differ considerably in their oxygen content from mixed venous blood.'

24 hours after a major operation, the patient is cyanosed. Arterial blood is analysed with the following results: P_{O_2} 105 mm Hg, P_{CO_2} 55 mm Hg, pH = 7.54. It follows that:-

A. the patient is breathing an oxygen-enriched atmosphere
B. respiratory alkalosis is present
C. metabolic alkalosis is present
D. bronchopulmonary segmental collapse may be the cause of the cyanosis
E. cardiac output is normal.

105

55 $\rightarrow$ acid

7.54 $\rightarrow$ alk.

T
F
T
F

$$ H = pk + \log \left\{ \frac{HCO_3}{H_2CO_3} \right\} = 20 \cdot \text{ at } 7.4$$
6.1

Answers overleaf

R10 Answers

A. TRUE This answer requires consideration of the gas tensions in this patient's alveolar gas and arterial blood. Since Pa_{CO_2} is 55 mm Hg and the measurable gradient of CO_2-tension between arterialised blood and alveolar gas is zero (because CO_2 is so freely diffusible), the alveolar carbon dioxide tension Pa_{CO_2} must be 55 mm Hg also. The simple version of the alveolar gas equation states that alveolar oxygen tension, Pa_{O_2}, is given by the expression

$$Pa_{O_2} = Pi_{O_2} - \frac{Pa_{CO_2}}{R}$$

where Pi_{O_2} is the inspired oxygen tension, R the respiratory quotient. The normal value of R is about 0.85 and that of Pi_{O_2} about 150, i.e. (21% × (760-47)) mm Hg, where 21% is the fractional concentration of oxygen in the inspired gas, 760 is the barometric pressure and 47 the vapour pressure of saturated water vapour at 37°C. Substitution in the equation gives a value of Pa_{O_2} of 85 mm Hg. Even if R is as high as the maximum possible, i.e. 1, Pa_{O_2} can only reach 95 mm Hg. So if Pa_{O_2} is as high as 105 mm Hg, the patient must be breathing an oxygen-enriched atmosphere.

B. & C. FALSE and TRUE An arterial carbon dioxide tension (Pa_{CO_2}) greater than the normal 44 mm Hg defines respiratory acidosis, i.e. a tendency towards acidity due to the accumulation of carbon dioxide due to underventilation. The patient's respiratory acidosis would, if the metabolic component of acid-base balance were normal, result in the pH of the arterial plasma being more acid than normal, i.e. less than 7.4. The higher value of 7.54 actually present means that there must be a metabolic alkalosis outweighing the respiratory acidosis.

D. FALSE When bronchopulmonary segmental collapse causes cyanosis, the mechanism is that in the areas of collapse, mixed venous blood is passing through non-aerated alveoli and hence contributing blood with a low oxygen content and partial pressure to the systemic arterial blood. In other words, the Pa_{O_2} should be low enough to explain the cyanosis. In the present patient, however, the Pa_{O_2} is within normal limits and so bronchopulmonary segmental collapse cannot be the factor producing cyanosis.

E. FALSE With Pa_{O_2} within normal limits, the only possible cause for the blood in the tissues to have a high concentration of reduced haemoglobin is that the blood is staying longer in contact with the tissues than normal, and so is losing more oxygen to the tissues than normal. This situation occurs when the blood flow through the tissues is reduced, i.e. when cardiac output is low.

140

NOTE: The simple form of the Alveolar Gas Equation used here is derived from the facts that nitrogen is inert and neither leaves nor enters the respiratory gases, that there is virtually no carbon dioxide in inspired gas and that the volume (and therefore partial pressure) of any CO_2 in the alveoli is related to the volume reduction (and therefore partial pressure reduction) of oxygen from the level of inspired gas by the fraction known as the respiratory quotient:

$$\frac{O_2 \text{ produced}}{O_2 \text{ used}} = R,$$

$$\text{so } O_2 \text{ used} = \frac{CO_2 \text{ produced}}{R}$$

2. CARDIOVASCULAR AND BLOOD

C1 Questions

With respect to capillaries:-

A. hydrostatic pressure at the arterial end is greater than the effective osmotic pressure of the plasma proteins
B. hydrostatic pressure at the venous end is smaller than the effective osmotic pressure of the plasma proteins
C. calibre can vary continuously through the range fully patent — fully collapsed
D. over-distended capillaries are more permeable to plasma proteins than normal capillaries
E. in vigorously exercising muscle practically all the capillaries are fully open.

C2 Questions

In the normal ECG tracing:-

A. the P-wave is due to arterial excitation
B. the upper limit of the normal P—R interval is 0.1 sec.
C. the QRS complex represents ventricular excitation
D. the R-wave may be inverted in lead I and upright in lead III
E. the T-wave occurs during ventricular systole.

Answers overleaf

C1 Answers

A. TRUE   Thus nett movement of water and electrolytes at the arterial end of the capillary is out into the interstitial fluid.

B. TRUE   Thus nett movement of water and electrolytes at the venous end of the capillary is back into the capillary.

C. FALSE   A capillary is either fully open or fully collapsed—or else over-distended (see D). The factors deciding the patency of a capillary are not fully understood.

D. TRUE   For example, in the situation of high venous pressure due to strangulation of a vascular pedicle, the back-pressure of the capillaries over-distends them and there is a tendency for protein-rich liquid to exude into the strangulated tissues.

E. TRUE   The local vast increases in hydrogen ion and other products of active metabolism are thought to produce this effect.

C2 Answers

A. TRUE   The P-wave represents the spread of the electrical impulse from the sinu-atrial node through both atria.

B. FALSE   The P—R interval does not normally exceed 0.22 sec.

C. TRUE   The QRS complex represents the activation of the whole ventriculr mass.

D. TRUE   Right- (and left-) axis deviation can result from an altered orientation of a normal heart. Thus a heart lying more vertically than normal produces right-axis deviation (R-waves inverted in lead I and upright in lead III), whilst a heart lying more horizontally produces left-axis deviation.

E. TRUE   The T-wave occupies much of the second half of ventricular systole.

During the process of normal haemostasis:-

A. platelets adhere to all water-wettable surfaces
B. platelets adhere to any damaged vascular endothelial surface
C. platelet-cohesion, i.e. the adherence of platelets to each other, can take place in the absence of calcium ions
D. the largest contributor to the strength of the mature blood clot is fibrin
E. thrombin concentrations remain high in the vicinity of a formed clot for about one hour.

Answers overleaf

C3 Answers

A. FALSE   In general, platelets do adhere to water-wettable surfaces, but this is not universally true. Indeed, there is one common water-wettable surface that platelets do not adhere to, and just as well! — the normal vascular endothelium.

B. TRUE   This reaction is immediate, but the mechanism is unknown.

C. FALSE   Adhesion to a damaged or foreign surface is the first step, and after this has occurred the platelets undergo changes in the presence of calcium ions and ADP that result in their sticking to each other (cohesion). The calcium ions are essential; indeed, if calcium ions are removed from the region of coherent platelets the latter become re-dispersed, apparently normal.

D. FALSE   Fibrin only forms 0.2 per cent of the weight of blood clot although its interlaced adhesive fibres are responsible for most of the strength of the clot.

E. FALSE   All the active agents involved in blood-clotting, including thrombin, vanish within a few minutes of the completion of the clot. The mechanism is unknown, but this feature of normal clotting is crucial to the prevention of spontaneous thrombosis.

Haemolytic disease of the newborn:-

F

anti A
anti B

A. due to ABO incompatibility never occurs if the mother is group O
B. due to ABO incompatibility is almost as common as that due to rhesus incompatibility
C. affects rhesus positive infants born to rhesus negative mothers F
D. occurs at least to some extent in about 15 per cent of all pregnancies F
E. due to rhesus incompatibility can be prevented by injecting, shortly after parturition, mothers who are at risk of immunisation with anti-D antibody.

Rh+ve — presence N Ag
Rh-ve — no Ag

Ag→ mum → Ag in mum →bake

Answers overleaf

C4 Answers

A. FALSE In practice, ABO incompatibility haemolytic disease occurs only in cases where the mother is group O, because individuals of group O make more anti-A and anti-B antibody than do individuals of other groups.

B. TRUE The incompatibility is usually only apparent on serological testing, or at most clinically mild, because the infant's A and/or B antigens are immature at birth and widely distributed in all tissues except the brain. By contrast, the Rh antigens are fully developed at birth and present only in red cells so that the latter bear the full force of the attack from any maternal antibodies.

C. TRUE If the Rh-negative mother has been previously immunized by transfusion or an earlier pregnancy her anti-Rh antibodies cross the placenta and attack the Rh-positive cells of the foetus.

D. FALSE The figure of 15 per cent represents the percentage of women who are Rh-negative and therefore theoretically at risk. However, the infant will be Rh-negative if the father is Rh-negative, and has a 50% chance of also being Rh-negative if the father is heterozygous Rh-Negative (Dd). Only if the father is homozygous Rh-positive (DD) will the infant definitely be Rh-positive. Even if the infant is indeed Rh-positive, the chance that the mother will have a transplacental haemorrhage from the foetal circulation is only about 5%, and the chance that immunization results from that haemorrhage is probably only about 15% of that 5%. Haemolytic disease of the newborn due to rhesus incompatibility is a rare disease.

E. TRUE IgG anti-D, injected into the mother within 24-48 hours of delivery, clears her circulation of Rh-positive cells before they can produce immunization.

148

The sinu-atrial node:-

A. is nervous tissue

B. lies in the right atrial wall near the entrance of the *superior* vena cava

C. has an intrinsic rhythm of activity of 300 – 400 beats per minute

D. produces a maximal contraction of the atria or none at all

E. must function normally to produce effective atrial contractions if adequate cardiac output is to be maintained.

Answers overleaf

C5 Answers

A. FALSE   Histologically, the sinu-atrial (SA) node is specialized myocardial tissue.

B. TRUE

C. FALSE   The intrinsic rhythm of the SA node is 50 – 150 beats per minute. However, abnormal centres in the atrium that develop in certain disease states (atrial flutter) may have an intrinsic rate as high as 300 – 400 beats per minute.

D. TRUE   This is an example of the 'all or none' law that applies to all myocardial tissue.

E. FALSE   Even when there is no effective atrial contraction (e.g. in atrial fibrillation) an adequate cardiac output can be maintained.

In running a blood transfusion service it is important to bear in mind the physiological principle that:-

A. the lower age limit for accepting habitual donors is 15 years   F

B. pregnancy is not a contraindication to routine donation   F

C. regular donations may be accepted from any male donor as often   T
   as every 3 months

D. blood should be stored at 0°C to reduce the rate at which ageing   F
   occurs

E. crossmatching of the donor's cells should be performed with the   T
   recipient's plasma.

Answers overleaf

C6 Answers

A. & B. FALSE The absorbable iron content of a normal, meat-containing diet is sufficient to keep an adult male in balance. Any extra demands on the iron supplies in the body result in iron deficiency unless the intake of iron is supplemented. Extra demands include normal growth in childhood, the requirements of the foetus in pregnancy, and blood loss. Adult men require 10 mg iron per day, adult women 12 mg (because of the blood loss through menstruation), pregnant women 15 mg, and children aged 13 – 20 years 15 mg per day. Thus it would be physiologically inadvisable to accept habitual donors from the groups of youths aged 15 – 20 years, or from pregnant females.

C. TRUE Blood contains 0.5 mg iron per ml, so the usual blood donation causes a loss of about 200 mg iron. In a man, the normal small excess of dietary intake over faecal and urinary losses would be adequate to make good this loss in three months.

D. FALSE Blood is stored at a temperature of 4°C to lower the rate of the metabolic processes that age the stored red cells and reduce their suitability for transfusion. The temperature of 0°C would introduce a risk of freezing of the water in the red blood cells: the expansion when it becomes ice would burst the red cells and the consequent haemolysis would be likely to cause serious or even fatal reaction when the blood was subsequently transfused.

E. When blood is transfused, haemolysis due to incompatibility is possible either if the donor's cells are agglutinated by the recipient's plasma, or if the recipient's cells are agglutinated by the donor's plasma. In practice, the donor's plasma is so rapidly diluted by the recipient's plasma after transfusion that any effect of the donor's plasma on the recipient's cells can usually be discounted. The important consideration is, does the recipient's plasma agglutinate the donor's cells.

During the cardiac cycle:-

A. the filling of the right atrium is reduced by inspiration   T
B. the filling of the left atrium is increased by expiration
C. early in ventricular diastole, ventricular filling is rapid
D. just before the end of ventricular diastole, ventricular filling is   T
   rapid
E. the spontaneous rhythm of the ventricles, if not stimulated from
   the atria, is 60 − 80 beats per minute.   F

The arteriolar smooth muscle:-

A. is mainly controlled by nervous impulses mediated by the
   parasympathetic nervous system
B. responds only to noradrenaline
C. is the main factor determining peripheral resistance
D. of the cerebral circulation is particularly responsive to impulses
   received via autonomic nerves
E. contracts in response to an increased local concentration of
   histamine.

Answers overleaf

C7 Answers

A. FALSE   Inspiration, i.e. the enlargement of the musculo-skeletal thoracic cavity, reduces intra-pleural pressure and so increases the venous return to the right atrium via the venae cavae.

B. TRUE   Expiration, i.e. the reduction in size of the thorax, expels extra blood from the lungs via the pulmonary veins into the left atrium.

C. TRUE   This is the early rapid filling phase, produced by rapid relaxation of the ventricles after the end of ventricular systole and the opening of the mitral and tricuspid valves.

D. TRUE   This is the phase of contraction of the atria, with forcible propulsion into the ventricles of the blood still left in their cavities.

E. FALSE   The idio-ventricular rhythm (seen for example in complete heart block) is 30 − 40 beats per minute.

C8 Answers

A. FALSE   It is the *sympathetic* nervous system that is the main controller of the calibre of arterioles.

B. FALSE   Noradrenaline is the transmitter of sympathetic *vasoconstrictor* impulses, but some arterioles possess a *vasodilator* sympathetic innervation (either with or without a vasoconstrictor innervation). The chemical transmitter of such vasodilator nerve fibres is acetyl choline.

C. TRUE

D. FALSE   There is no significant venoconstriction in the cerebral blood vessels when there is a fall in blood pressure or heart rate. This is an important factor in maintaining cerebral perfusion when the cardiac output falls.

E. FALSE   Histamine dilates arterioles and is thereby responsible for the headache, and flushing of the skin, characteristic of the response to histamine.

3. GASTROINTESTINAL TRACT

Parotid gland salivary secretion:-

A. ceases during sleep
B. is secreted at a rate that is hormone-dependent
C. increases when the subject thinks of food
D. contains more mucus than saliva from the submandibular gland
E. contains more amylase than saliva from the submandibular gland.

Saliva contains:-

A. a fixed concentration of sodium ions
B. a concentration of chloride ions that increases with the rate of secretion
C. a concentration of potassium higher than that in plasma
D. a concentration of iodide ions higher than that in the plasma
E. the blood group A, B and O agglutinogens (in those individuals who secrete them) in the same concentration as in blood.

Answers overleaf

G1 Answers

A. TRUE   There is a so-called 'resting' secretion during the day, but this low rate of secretion seems to be due to minor stimuli that occur during wakefulness even in the absence of food, movement of the jaws, etc. During sleep all secretion from the parotid ceases.

B. FALSE   No hormones have been found to affect cells involved in the primary secretion.

C. Unlike the situation in dogs, no such direct conditioned reflex can be demonstrated in man. An individual often *says* that his 'mouth is watering' under these circumstances, but since objective measurement shows no excess salivation the explanation must be that he becomes more aware of his resting secretion.

D. FALSE   The parotid secretion is mainly serous, the submandibular, mucous.

E. TRUE   Amylase concentrations are greater in the parotid secretion than in the secretions from any of the other salivary glands, including the unnamed ones.

G2 Answers

A. FALSE   The $[Na^+]$ is very low in resting secretion $(1-5 \text{ mmol/l})$ but rises with increasing rates of secretion to levels as high as 100 mmol/l.

B. TRUE   The $[Cl^-]$ is similarly low $(1-5 \text{ mmol/l})$ in resting secretion, but rises with increasing rates of secretion to levels of about 70 mmol/l.

C. TRUE   The $[K^+]$ is less dependent than $[Na^+]$ or $[Cl^-]$ on secretion rate, but it is always greater than the concentration in plasma, in the range $10-30 \text{ mmol/l}$.

D. TRUE   The salivary glands extract iodide from the plasma and excrete the ion in the saliva at a much greater concentration.

E. FALSE   In the 80% of individuals who secrete the blood group agglutinogens, these substances are present in the saliva in concentrations up to 100 times those in blood.

Intrinsic factor is:-

A. a peptide with a chain of 17 amino acids
B. secreted by the same cells that secrete hydrochloric acid
C. secreted in just sufficient quantities to perform its function
D. essential for the absorption of vitamin B_{12} (cyanocobalamin)
E. likely to be secreted at a very low rate if hypochlorhydria due to chronic gastritis is present.

Gastrin:-

A. is a polypeptide
B. exists in the circulating plasma as a single molecular species
C. is elaborated in 'G-cells' that are confined to the antral region of the stomach
D. stimulates secretion of pepsinogen more strongly than secretion of hydrogen ions
E. is best measured by a biological assay via its effect on gastric acid secretion in small mammals.

Answers overleaf

G3 Answers

A. FALSE   Intrinsic factor (IF) is a glycoprotein with a molecular weight of about 55,000.

B. TRUE   The parietal cell secretes both IF and hydrochloric acid (in the human).

C. FALSE   IF is secreted in great excess compared with the amount required. The surplus is inactivated by hydrochloric acid.

D. TRUE   No absorption of vitamin B_{12} is possible in the absence of IF.

E. FALSE   The effect of gastritis on the ability of the parietal cells to secrete hydrochloric acid is usually much greater than the effect on their ability to secrete IF. Therefore, the secretion of IF continues at relatively normal rates long after the secretion of hydrochloric acid has become markedly depressed.

G4 Answers

A. TRUE

B. FALSE   There are at least two biologically active forms of circulating gastrin: G 17, which contains a chain of 17 amino acids, and G 34, which contains 34 amino acids. There are also larger and smaller molecules of the same family, but the biological importance of these is doubtful.

C. FALSE   The cells that elaborate gastrin are called G-cells, but they are not confined to the antral region of the stomach. Quite apart from the fact that a sparse scattering of G-cells has been demonstrated in the parietal cell area of the stomach, G-cells also occur in the duodenum and (in decreasing proportion) along the ·proximal jejunum, and these G-cells at distal sites may be involved in the intestinal phase of gastric secretion.

D. FALSE   The principal effect of gastrin is to increase acid production, although there is a weaker effect on pepsinogen production.

E. FALSE   The biological assay is time-consuming and subject to many errors—in particular, the variable response of individual animals to the same dose of gastrin; in practice it has been superseded by radioimmunoassay (see Q E11 p 19).

Fasting plasma concentrations of (physiologically active) gastrin are:-

A. higher in men than in women
B. abnormally high in most patients with duodenal ulcer
C. abnormally low in most patients with gastric ulcer
D. abnormally high in most patients after vagotomy for duodenal ulcer
E. abnormally high in individuals exhibiting achlorhydria.

Inhibitors of gastric acid secretion include:-

A. pancreatic glucagon
B. acidification of the duodenum
C. vasoactive intestinal polypeptide (VIP)
D. protein in the duodenum
E. calcium ions.

Answers overleaf

G5 Answers

A. FALSE   There is no sex difference in fasting plasma gastrin concentrations.

B. C. D. & E. FALSE, FALSE, TRUE and TRUE   The key to understanding these relationships is that gastrin production is depressed by a high acidity (hydrogen ion concentration) and stimulated by a low acidity in the antrum. Patients with duodenal ulcer have a tendency to be hypersecretors of gastric acid compared with normal subjects, so that there is a tendency for fasting plasma gastrin to be low (the effect is not sufficiently marked to be statistically significant in most patients with a duodenal ulcer). Patients with a gastric ulcer tend, if anything to secrete *less* acid than normal subjects and there is a definite tendency for their fasting plasma gastrin values to be high. After an effective vagotomy, the ability of the stomach to secrete acid is reduced and so fasting serum gastrin concentration rises. The same effect is seen to a much more pronounced level in complete achlorhydria—such subjects may have gastrin levels twenty times the upper limit for the normal population.

G6 Answers

A. TRUE   This effect can be demonstrated in experiments on animals, but there is no good evidence that it is of physiological importance in man.

B. TRUE   The mechanism is not entirely known: it is partly via the vagus, since the effect of truncal vagotomy is to reduce the inhibitory power of duodenal acidification, but other mechanisms certainly exist as well. They may involve other nervous pathways, e.g. the sympathetic, or else a humoral mechanism.

C. TRUE   This hormone powerfully inhibits gastric secretion when liberated in excess from tumours ('Vipomas') that usually occur in the pancreas. The other important effect of this hormone is to produce watery diarrhoea. The physiological role of VIP is not clear.

D. FALSE   It is the presence in the duodenum of fat, or a solution of high osmotic pressure, that inhibits gastric secretion, probably via a hormonal intermediary.

E. FALSE   There is, if anything, a slight tendency for an increase in calcium ion concentration in the plasma to *increase* gastric secretion in normal subjects.

Features suggestive of the Zollinger-Ellison syndrome (peptic ulcer diathesis due to a gastrin-secreting tumour of the pancreas) include:-

A. basal gastric secretion in the normal range
B. a high ratio ($>$0.6) of basal to maximal secretion
C. inhibition of gastric secretion by calcium ions
D. inhibition of gastrin release by calcium ions
E. stimulation of gastrin release by secretin.

The rate at which a liquid meal leaves the stomach is:-

A. proportional to the volume of the stomach contents
B. greater in the upright than in the supine position
C. greater if the meal contains fat
D. smaller if the meal is 5% glucose than if it is 50% glucose
E. smaller if vagotomy and a drainage procedure (such as gastroenterostomy or pyloroplasty) has been performed.

Answers overleaf

G7 Answers

A. False These autonomous tumours usually release large quantities of gastrin into the circulation all the time. In consequence, basal levels of gastric secretion are usually higher than normal. (This effect is not always present: occasionally the release of excess gastrin is intermittent).

B. TRUE Because of the usual increased gastrin drive, 'basal' secretion usually approaches fully stimulated secretion. The ratio of 0.6 has been determined empirically.

C. FALSE Calcium ions show a slight tendency to stimulate gastric secretion even in normal subjects; in patients with this syndrome the effect is much greater.

D. & E. FALSE and TRUE The stimulatory effect of calcium, ions on gastric secretion in patients with this syndrome acts via an effect promoting the release of gastrin from the tumour. Intravenous injections of secretin have a similar effect.

G8 Answers

A. TRUE Because the rate of emptying at any moment is proportional to the volume present in the stomach at that moment, the decay curve of a meal in the stomach is semiexponential—the logarithm of the amount of meal left in the stomach is related linearly to time.

B. FALSE Gastric emptying accelerates when the patient lies down.

C. FALSE When the fat reaches the duodenum it stimulates a mixed hormonal/vagal mechanism that brakes the rate of stomach emptying.

D. FALSE There are receptors sensitive to osmotic pressure in the duodenum. The 5% glucose meal is isotonic and will empty at maximal rate, but osmotically stronger (and weaker) solutions will empty more slowly.

E. FALSE Vagotomy may temporarily slow gastric emptying, but its long term effect, even if the innervation of the antrum is preserved (by, for example, the operation of proximal gastric—highly selective—vagotomy) is to *increase* the rate of gastric emptying in some patients or to leave it unchanged in others. Pyloroplasty destroys and gastroenterostomy by-passes the pyloric braking mechanism, and so the combined effect of vagotomy and a drainage procedure is a definite tendency towards accelerating gastric emptying.

In patients who have undergone gastric surgery, factors involved in the pathogenesis of early post-prandial symptoms of the dumping syndrome include:-

A. fall in plasma volume
B. rise in blood glucose concentration
C. increase in rate of gastric emptying
D. fall in plasma protein concentration
E. excessive rise in plasma insulin concentration.

The small intestine:-

A. in life is about 3 m (9 ft.) long
B. lining cells (enterocytes) have the fastest turnover rate of any cells in the body
C. produces, preponderantly among the immunoglobulins, IgG.
D. Paneth cells have no known function
E. argentaffin cells reabsorb bile salts.

Answers overleaf

G9 Answers

A. TRUE   The fall in plasma volume is not the only factor, but it is clearly implicated. After a standard glucose meal (150 – 200 ml. 50% solution), patients with a fall in plasma volume of less than 8% never complain of dumping symptoms, patients with a fall greater than 17% always complain of such symptoms, while patients with the clinical syndrome always show a fall in plasma volume of 9% or greater.

B. FALSE   The blood glucose concentration does tend to rise higher in patients with the syndrome than in those without, but the same levels of blood glucose produced by an intravenous infusion of glucose never produce the symptoms.

C. TRUE   There is a good positive correlation between fast gastric emptying, the associated fall in plasma volume, and the symptoms.

D. FALSE   The plasma volume shrinks because it loses water and electrolytes into the lumen of the gut (as a result of the osmotic attraction of the rapidly emptied glucose meal)—but not plasma proteins, so the concentration of these rises.

E. FALSE   The *late* post-prandial symptoms (two hours after the meal) sometimes known as late dumping are hypoglycaemic in origin and result from an overshoot of insulin production in response to the hyperglycaemia produced by the rapidly emptying meal.

G10 Answers

A. TRUE   Anatomical textbooks usually quote a figure of 7 m. (20 ft), but such measurements have been made in cadavers; the tonic contraction of the longitudinal muscle produces the smaller figure in the living subject.

B. TRUE   The whole process of formation of the enterocyte at the base of a crypt, migration on to the surface, and then further movement upwards along a villus to its tip where the cell is shed, takes only 4 days.

C. FALSE   The immunoglobin mainly produced is IgA, as is the case with most other external secretions, and in contrast with the limited proportion (about 15%) of IgA present in plasma.

D. TRUE

E. FALSE   The function of the argentaffin cells is to secrete 5-hydroxytryptamine.

164

Factors definitely increasing small bowel motility include:-

A. truncal vagotomy
B. gastroenterostomy with or without partial gastrectomy
C. sympathectomy
D. thyroxine excess
E. 5-hydroxytryptamine.

Recognised complications of the excision of the terminal metre (3 ft) of the ileum (with preservation of the ileocaecal valve) include:-

A. a lag type of glucose tolerance curve
B. iron deficiency anaemia
C. low concentrations of folate in the erythrocytes
D. gallstones
E. malabsorption of fat.

Answers overleaf

G11 Answers

A. FALSE There may be some increased segmentation in the small bowel, particularly the ileum, but on the other hand transit time is increased in some patients, at least temporarily.

B. TRUE When the pylorus is destroyed or by-passed, there is usually increased peristalsis in the jejunum, in association with an increased rate of gastric emptying and accompanying intestinal distension.

C. FALSE Sympathectomy has no clear-cut effect.

D. TRUE Diarrhoea is a typical symptom of thyrotoxicosis.

E. TRUE Diarrhoea is a typical feature of the carcinoid syndrome, in which 5-HT is intermittently secreted from a tumour of argentaffin cells. 5-HT is released from cells in the intestinal wall when the bowel is distended, and increases the frequency of peristalsis locally.

G12 Answers

A. FALSE A lag curve is one in which the blood glucose concentration rises rapidly to a high level, and then falls rapidly with an overshoot to hypoglycaemic levels. It results from rapid absorption of glucose and an overswing in insulin production. When small bowel absorption is impaired by excision of a significant proportion of the bowel, a flat glucose tolerance curve results.

B. FALSE The main sites of absorption of iron are in the duodenum and upper jejunum.

C. FALSE The main site of absorption of folate is the jejunum.

D. TRUE The entero-hepatic recirculation of bile salts is normally maintained by the reabsorption in the distal ileum of most of the bile salts reaching the duodenum in the bile. The consequent strain on the synthesis of bile salts and contraction of the bile salt pool reduces their solubilizing effects on cholesterol in the bile and a consequent tendency towards the precipitation of gallstones.

E. TRUE The mechanism is the same as in D above, i.e., the contraction of the bile salts pool and reduction of their solubilizing effect on luminal fat.

Deficiency of the group of enzymes known as maltase in the brush border of the cells lining the intestinal lumen:-

A. does not prevent the hydrolyis of maltose, which can be hydrolysed in the intestinal lumen by pancreatic amylase
B. reduces the rate of absorption of ingested glucose
C. results in an increased bulk of the stool
D. results in increased passage of flatus
E. results in lack of absorption of lactose.

Ingested protein:-

A. is almost completely absorbed
B. is absorbed mostly in the terminal ileum
C. is very poorly absorbed in the absence of gastric peptic activity
D. can be absorbed only after hydrolysis to individual amino acids
E. after hydrolysis to individual amino acids is absorbed by active transport systems.

Answers overleaf

G13 Answers

A. FALSE   Pancreatic α-amylase takes the hydrolysis of starch only to the stage of maltose, maltotriose, and α-limit dextrin.

B. FALSE   The only substrates whose hydrolysis is catalysed by maltase are maltose and maltotriose.

C. TRUE   The increased osmotic pressure of the bowel contents resulting from the lack of absorption of maltose and maltotriose results in an increased water content of the stool.

D. TRUE   The unabsorbed disaccharides are metabolized by bacterial action in the colon to produce organic acids, and further fermentation of these produces carbon dioxide.

E. FALSE   See B above.

G14 Answers

A. TRUE   Absorption is at least 95% complete (only 1 – 2 g is lost in the faeces each 24 hours, and most of this is derived from secretions and surface detritus).

B. FALSE   Most protein absorption occurs in the upper two-thirds of the small intestine.

C. FALSE   Gastric pepsin is relatively unimportant: most of the hydrolysis of proteins results from the activity, in the alkaline milieu of the duodenum, of pancreatic trypsin.

D. FALSE   Most absorption does occur in the form of individual amino acids, but some oligopeptides (mainly dipeptides) can be absorbed.

E. TRUE   The carrier mechanisms involved are (like that of glucose) sodium-linked, and are more effective for the laevo-rotatory than the dextro-rotatory isomers.

The absorption of fat:-

A. from the diet is more than 95% complete
B. mostly occurs in the terminal metre (3 ft) of the ileum
C. is impaired by excision of the terminal metre (3 ft) of the ileum
D. takes place to a substantial extent in the form of solubilized triglycerides
E. into the lymphatics occurs mostly in the form of free fatty acids.

Bile salts:-

A. are formed in the liver
B. form a pool much greater in size than the amount excreted daily via the bile into the duodenum
C. form micelles when exposed to the alkalinity of the duodenal lumen
D. in pure micellar form can solubilize the fat-soluble vitamins
E. inhibit the absorption of water and sodium in the colon.

Answers overleaf

G15 Answers

A. TRUE   A daily load of up to 200 g can be thus efficiently absorbed.

B. FALSE   Absorption of fat takes place mostly in the distal half of the duodenum and the proximal half of the jejunum.

C. TRUE   Despite the answer to B above, resection of the terminal ileum produces steatorrhoea by preventing the reabsorption of bile salts, thus reducing the bile salt pool and the consequent availability of bile salts in the upper small bowel where they are needed to promote fat absorption.

D. FALSE   Triglycerides cannot be solubilized by incorporation in the bile salt micelles; they must be converted to monoglycerides and free fatty acids.

E. FALSE   The monoglycerides and free fatty acids absorbed into the mucosal villous cells are reconstituted into triglycerides, the latter are incorporated into chylomicrons, and these are extruded into the lymphatics.

G16 Answers

A. TRUE   They result from the oxidation of cholesterol.

B. FALSE   The excretion of bile salts into the duodenum, about 20 – 30 g daily, is much greater than the bile salt pool of 1 – 3 g. Even with a single meal, the bile salt secretion may greatly exceed the size of the pool.

C. FALSE   The micelles (polymolecular aggregates) are formed when the concentration of bile salts exceeds a critical level: pH is not an important factor.

D. FALSE   Simple micelles of bile salts cannot solubilize certain monoglycerides, cholesterol and the fat-soluble vitamins. However, after incorporation into the micelles of other monoglycerides and fatty acids, the resultant mixed micelles can solubilize these substances.

E. TRUE   When bile salts reach the colon in significant amounts, they provoke a watery diarrhoea—partly by this effect on absorption and partly by an irritant action on the mucosa.

The absorption of water from the alimentary tract:-

A. is mainly a passive process
B. occurs to a marked extent in the stomach
C. occurs mostly in the colon
D. is modified by changes in secretion rate of aldosterone
E. is hindered by a high osmotic pressure in the luminal contents

Absorption of calcium from the digestive tract:-

A. takes place mostly in the proximal jejunum
B. is prevented by the presence of small amounts of phytic acid in the diet, even when an excess of calcium is ingested
C. is facilitated by the presence of fat in the food
D. can be reversed (i.e. calcium is secreted from the blood into the bowel lumen) when plasma calcium concentration is raised by a calcium infusion
E. is about as rapid as that of sodium.

Answers overleaf

G17 Answers

A. TRUE   Water absorption seems to occur by passive diffusion in response to osmotic gradients across the bowel wall. These gradients are produced by absorption of glucose and electrolytes in the small bowel, and of sodium in the large bowel.

B. FALSE   The amount of absorption in the stomach is negligible.

C. FALSE   Eight or nine litres of secretions of the upper alimentary tract, plus the water of the diet, are presented to the small intestine daily: less than 1 litre is left unabsorbed to enter the large bowel, which then absorbs all but 100 ml—the water content of faeces.

D. TRUE   Increased aldosterone secretion, for example in states of sodium deficiency, results in an increased reabsorption of sodium in the colon and this is accompanied by an increased passive reabsorption of water.

E. TRUE   This is the mechanism of the diarrhoea produced by the non-absorbable saline purgatives, and by the rapid entry of hyperosmotic food solutions into the jejunum in the dumping syndrome: the high osmotic pressure in the lumen attracts water from the circulation into the lumen.

G18 Answers

A. TRUE

B. FALSE   Phytic acid produces insoluble (and non-absorbable) calcium phytate: when all the phytic acid has been precipitated, the excess calcium is absorbed.

C. FALSE   Fatty acids form insoluble calcium salts (soaps).

D. FALSE   The shift of calcium ions across the intestinal mucosa is virtually one-way.

E. FALSE   Sodium is absorbed at a speed fifty times that of calcium absorption. Intestinal hurry is therefore an important factor producing malabsorption of calcium.

Vitamins that, when ingested in excessive amounts, can produce harmful effects include:-

A. Vitamin B_{12} (cyanocobalamin)
B. Vitamin B_6 (pyridoxal)
C. Vitamin C (ascorbic acid)
D. Vitamin A
E. Vitamin D.

Factors helping to maintain ano-rectal continence include:-

A. continuous resting tone in the internal anal sphincter
B. the ability to maintain voluntary contraction of the external anal sphincter indefinitely
C. the upright posture
D. the somatic sensation in the epithelium of the anal canal
E. cortical inhibition of the urge to defecate.

Answers overleaf

G19 Answers

A. B. & C. FALSE   All three are water soluble vitamins which are not stored to any significant extent in the body, but are excreted when plasma levels exceed the renal threshold.

D. TRUE   Hypervitaminosis has been described in children: the abnormalities produced are a dry, rough skin, polyarthritis and an enlarged liver.

E. TRUE   Hypervitaminosis D causes widespread calcification in many soft tissues, including kidneys and lungs.

G20 Answers

A. TRUE   This is the most important single factor in the preservation of continence.

B. FALSE   The external anal sphincter has a low resting tone, not important in itself in preserving continence, since the anal canal is normally empty. When material enters the upper anal canal, the resulting distension causes a very temporary increase in external sphincter tone, and this can be further augmented by voluntary effort for 40 – 60 seconds only.

C. TRUE   Flexing the hips reduces the 80° angle between the rectum and the anal canal, and is almost an essential preliminary to defecation.

D. TRUE   This somatic sensation in the anal canal is important: it enables the subject to distinguish between solid, liquid and gas entering the anal canal so that appropriate decisions can be made about permitting, or not permitting, the release of the material. See E below.

E. TRUE   Normally the cortical centres make the decision between permitting defecation by inhibiting the external sphincter and encouraging abdominal and diaphragmatic action to increase intra-abdominal pressure: or alternatively to increase voluntary contraction of the external sphincter, whereupon the urge to defecate gradually passes off.

During the excretion of bilirubin:-

A. conjugation of bilirubin is performed by microsomes of the smooth endoplasmic reticulum of liver cells
B. transport of bilirubin from the sites of formation to the liver occurs in erythrocytes
C. conjugation renders bilirubin lipid-soluble
D. conjugation is facilitated by phenobarbitone
E. bilirubin is conjugated with uridine diphosphate.

Cholestatic (as distinct from pre-hepatic) jaundice is characterised by:-

A. bilirubinuria
B. absence of urobilinogen from the urine
C. increased fragility of erythrocytes
D. deficiency of prothrombin
E. abnormal anatomy of the biliary apparatus as visualized by endoscopic retrograde cholangiopancreatography (ERCP).

Answers overleaf

G21 Answers

A. TRUE

B. FALSE   Transport to the liver takes place in plasma, where bilirubin is complexed with two acceptor proteins, labelled Y and Z.

C. FALSE   Bilirubin itself is lipid-soluble: conjugation converts it into a more water-soluble compound.

D. TRUE   This is an example of so-called *induction* of enzyme action by various drugs.

E. FALSE   The bilirubin is conjugated to glucuronic acid, derived from the substance uridine diphosphate glucuronic acid— UDPG, by the action of a particular one of the range of enzymes called glucuronyl transferases.

G22 Answers

A. TRUE   Cholestasis, i.e. an obstruction to the passage of conjugated bile from the site of conjugation in the hepatocytes towards the duodenum, results in a backflow of conjugated bilirubin into the blood. Conjugated bilirubin, unlike unconjugated (pre-hepatic) bilirubin, is water-soluble and is therefore excreted by the kidney to produce bilirubinuria. Pre-hepatic bile is not excreted in the urine—hence the term *acholuric jaundice*.

B. TRUE   In complete biliary obstruction, no bile reaches the lumen of the gastrointestinal tract, hence no urobilinogen is formed within the lumen, none is reabsorbed into the body, and so none is excreted in the urine. By contrast, in pre-hepatic jaundice bile is reaching the gastrointestinal tract and so urobilinogen (often in increased concentration) is excreted in the urine.

C. FALSE   Increased fragility of erythrocytes results in their rapid breakdown with a resultant pre-hepatic jaundice.

D. TRUE   If there is obstructive jaundice, bile salts also fail to reach the lumen of the duodenum and their solubilizing effect on fats is lost. This results in a reduced absorption of the fat-soluble vitamins including vitamin K, which is essential for the synthesis of prothrombin.

E. FALSE   Cholestasis may be due to obstruction in the major bile ducts but it may also occur at hepatocellular level, i.e. impaired transport of the conjugated form from the microsomes where conjugation takes place, across the cell to the bile canaliculi. Only if the obstruction is in the major bile duct will it be demonstrated by ERCP.

4. ENDOCRINOLOGY

E1 Questions

Endocrine glands and tissues related to the nervous system, i.e. either under ultimate hypothalamic control or derived from the neural crest, include the:-

A. follicular cells of the thyroid
B. kidney
C. gastrin-secreting cells of the alimentary tract
D. parafollicular cells of the thyroid
E. adrenal medulla.

E2 Questions

If serum thyroxine (T4) concentration is near the extremes (either the upper or the lower level) of normal range:-

A. a high concentration of protein-bound iodine confirms the thyrotoxicosis
B. measurement of the triiodothyronine concentration in plasma is usually helpful
C. if the T4 concentration is near the upper limit of normal the plasma concentration of thyroid-stimulating hormone (TSH) should be measured
D. if the T4 level is near the lower limit of normal T3 should be given in a large dose daily for one week and the measurement of T4 then repeated
E. if neither TSH measurement nor T4 measurement after T3 therapy gives an abnormal result, the patient cannot be thyrotoxic.

Answers overleaf

E1 Answers

A. TRUE   Thyroid-stimulating hormone (TSH) of the anterior pituitary stimulates the follicular cells of the thyroid and is itself under the control of the thyrotrophin-releasing hormone of the hypothalamus.

B. FALSE   The hormones of the kidney—renin, Vitamin D and erythropoietin—seem to be secreted independently of any nervous control and the cells concerned are not derived from the neural crest.

C. D. & E. ALL TRUE   Each tissue or organ is derived from the embryonic neural crest.

E2 Answers

A. FALSE   The plasma concentration of protein-bound iodine depends on so many factors other than the amount of circulating thyroxine (e.g. it is increased during pregnancy, by the administration of oestrogens, and in various low protein states), that it is not a reliable guide to the diagnosis of thyrotoxicosis.

B. FALSE   Thyrotoxicosis due to pure T3 excess is very rare (but see E below), so if the T4 concentration is equivocal the T3 concentration is likely to be equivocal too.

C. FALSE   The correct test to unmask equivocal thyrotoxicosis is the T3 suppression test (see D). T3 suppresses a moderately high, but normal, T4 level via the negative feed-back mechanism, but the raised T4 level of true thyrotoxicosis is autonomous.

D. FALSE   The correct test to confirm myxoedema is the measurement of TSH which should be high if the patient is myxoedematous, because of the negative feed-back mechanism.

E. FALSE   The rare condition of pure T3 thyrotoxicosis might be present.

Dietary iodine:-

A. is present particularly in fish
B. needs to amount to about 150 µg/day in order to maintain health
C. is absorbed mainly in the stomach and duodenum
D. is absorbed in the ionic form as iodide
E. is always below normal in the case of patients who have developed an iodine-deficiency goitre.

Oxytocin:-

A. has no known rôle in the male
B. is synthesised within the cells of the posterior lobe of the pituitary
C. stimulates the myoepithelial cells surrounding the alveoli and ducts of the lactating breast
D. is essential for the maintenance of pregnancy
E. secretion rate is increased by emotional stress.

Answers overleaf

E3 Answers

A. TRUE Fish and milk are the main dietary items rich in iodine, apart from iodized salt.

B. TRUE The output of iodine from the thyroid as T4 and T3 is about 70μg/day, and the figure 150μg/day is adequate to allow for wastage.

C. & D. FALSE and TRUE Iodine is mainly absorbed from the jejunum and ileum, in the form of iodide.

E. FALSE There may be certain chemical agents, known as goitrogens, present in the diet: they render some of the dietary iodine unavailable for absorption and iodine-deficiency goitre may result.

E4 Answers

A. TRUE

B. FALSE Like ADH, oxytocin is synthesized in the neurones of the hypothalamus, although mainly in the paraventricular rather than in the supraoptic nucleus.

C. TRUE It stimulates the ejection of milk from the nipple.

D. FALSE In high (pharmacological) doses, oxytocin stimulates the contraction of the pregnant uterus in women near term, and it is possible that it has a physiological action in the initiation of parturition, i.e. the termination of pregnancy.

E. FALSE The only known physiological stimuli for an increase in oxytocin secretion rate are suckling and vaginal distension during parturition (the Ferguson reflex).

Antidiuretic hormone (ADH) is:-

A. a protein
B. normally synthesized in the posterior lobe of the pituitary
C. very similar in structure to oxytocin
D. secreted at a lower rate when the osmotic pressure of the plasma rises
E. secreted at a rate independent of the concentration of all other hormones.

With regard to pituitary gonadotrophins in the female:-

A. follicle-stimulating hormone (FSH) stimulates the ovarian Graafian follicles to secrete oestrogens
B. luteinizing hormone (LH) is identical with prolactin
C. prolactin is responsible for the development of the female breast in puberty
D. prolactin is controlled by a hypothalamic inhibiting factor
E. total output in women as measured by 24-hour urinary excretion rates of 'total gonadotrophins' falls after the menopause.

Answers overleaf

E5 Answers

A. FALSE   ADH is a polypeptide composed of 8 amino acids.

B. FALSE   ADH is synthesized in the neurones of the hypothalamus, mainly in the supraoptic nucleus, and it passes down the axons into the stalk and posterior lobe, from which it is secreted into the circulation.

C. TRUE   Oxytocin also is a peptide containing 8 amino acids, 6 of which are identical in nature and sequence with the corresponding amino acids in ADH.

D. FALSE   When the osmotic pressure of the plasma rises, the hypothalamic osmoreceptors respond by increasing the rate of secretion of ADH, thus increasing the reabsorption of water in the distal convoluted tubules of the kidney and tending to restore the osmotic pressure of the plasma towards normal.

E. FALSE   The sensitivity of the ADH-secretion mechanism to changes in plasma osmotic pressure is depressed by a raised concentration of cortisol, increased by a lowered concentration of cortisol. Thus in cases of cortisol-deficiency (e.g. Addison's disease), the increased production of ADH resulting from hypersensitivity to the osmotic signal results in an inappropriate water retention and an abnormally low plasma osmotic pressure.

E6 Answers

A. TRUE   FSH causes the Graafian follicles to enlarge and secrete oestrogens.

B. FALSE   Prolactin used to be called luteotrophic hormone (LTH). LH, at mid-cycle, causes the follicle to rupture with release of the ovum and formation of the corpus luteum; for the functions of prolactin see C below.

C. FALSE   Development of the female breast at puberty is under ovarian control: prolactin is responsible for the initiation of lactation.

D. TRUE   Release of prolactin, unlike the other pituitary hormones under hypothalamic control, is inhibited rather than enhanced by its hypothalamic factor.

E. FALSE   After the menopause, the urinary excretion of gonadotrophins increases more than ten-fold, presumably due to the removal of a normal negative feedback control.

Thyroid-stimulating hormone (TSH):-

A. is produced by the posterior pituitary
B. is essential for the production of thyroxine by the thyroid gland
C. accelerates the rate at which the thyroid gland traps iodine from the blood
D. produced exophthalmos when its secretion rate is maximal
E. production rate is reduced when the plasma thyroxine concentration is high.

Adrenocorticotrophic hormone (ACTH):-

A. stimulates the adrenal cortex to secrete cortisol
B. is essential for the adrenal secretion of cortisol
C. increases the concentration of ascorbic acid in the adrenal cortex
D. is identical with melanophore-stimulating hormone (MSH)
E. is secreted at a constant rate.

Answers overleaf

E7 Answers

A. FALSE   TSH is produced in the anterior pituitary

B. FALSE   In the absence of TSH, the thyroid still synthesizes and releases thyroxine but at a much reduced rate.

C. TRUE   This is one of the many ways in which TSH increases the secretion-rate of thyroxine.

D. FALSE   Exophthalmos is produced by a different hormone, exophthalmos-producing substance (EPS). The two hormones are closely associated, and excess production of TSH may be accompanied by excess production of EPS, but they can nevertheless be separated.

E. TRUE   This is an example of a negative feed-back mechanism: the high concentration of thyroxine in the plasma damps down production of TSH by the pituitary.

E8 Answers

A. TRUE   The higher the plasma concentration of ACTH the greater the secretion rate of cortisol.

B. TRUE   In the absence of ACTH, there is virtually no demonstrable secretion of cortisol.

C. FALSE   ACTH causes a depletion of ascorbic acid in the cortex; this phenomenon forms the basis of one method of assaying ACTH.

D. FALSE   Pure ACTH has a slight melanophore-stimulating effect, but it is not the same substance as MSH.

E. FALSE   There is a circadian rhythm, so that in any 24-hour period resting values ranging between $10-300$ pg/l may be found.

Target glands and tissues for the hormones of the anterior pituitary include the:-

A. parafollicular cells of the thyroid
B. tubules of the testis
C. mammary gland
D. adrenal medulla
E. parathyroid glands.

Characteristic features of post-partum hypopituitarism include:-

A. normal lactation
B. permanent amenorrhoea
C. menopausal symptoms
D. severe sodium depletion
E. depigmentation of the areolae of the nipples.

Answers overleaf

E9 Answers

A. FALSE   Calcitonin release from the parafollicular cells is independent of the anterior pituitary.

B. TRUE   Follicle-stimulating hormone (FSH) stimulates development of the spermatic tubules.

C. TRUE   Prolactin is important for preparing the breast for lactation.

D. FALSE   Only the adrenal *cortex* is under pituitary control.

E. FALSE   Parathormone release is independent of the anterior pituitary.

E10 Answers

A. FALSE   Prolactin is essential to lactation.

B. TRUE   Absence of gonadotrophins causes permanent amenorrhoea. However—

C. FALSE   There are no menopausal symptoms.

D. FALSE   Although the secretion of aldosterone is not completely independent of the anterior pituitary, enough of this hormone is usually secreted to maintain a relatively normal water and sodium and potassium balance.

E. TRUE   Areolar pigmentation is under the control of melanophore-stimulating hormone (MSH) of the anterior pituitary and of oestrogens: both are lacking in severe hypopituitarism.

The radioimmunoassay of a hormone that is a protein:-

A. is not as accurate as chemical methods for measuring proteins
B. requires the presence of an auto-antibody to the hormone in the circulation of the subject whose hormone-concentration is being assayed
C. requires the injection of radioactively-labelled hormone into the subject
D. is usually much more sensitive than biological methods of assay
E. depends upon the reaction of the hormone *in vitro* with an antibody.

All hormones:-

A. act by stimulating the production of cyclic AMP
B. are used as a source of energy by their target organ
C. are secreted by tissues derived from the embryonic neural crest
D. permeate all the tissues of the body
E. are active in low concentrations (micromolar or less).

Answers overleaf

E11 Answers

A. FALSE There are no reliable chemical methods for measuring proteins.

B. FALSE See E.

C. FALSE See E.

D. TRUE Biological methods are subject to such errors due to variations in sensitivity between individual animals and to the generally low sensitivity of these techniques, that they are in practice confined to the measurement of a very few hormones, e.g. gonadotrophins. The radioimmunoassays are often a hundred times more sensitive than the corresponding bioassay.

E. TRUE An antibody to the hormone is raised in, say, a rabbit. The antibody is part of the rabbit gammaglobulin. The plasma sample being assayed is allowed to react with an excess of the gamma globulin, and its amount deduced from the amount of antibody left unreacted. The latter is determined by adding to the reaction-mixture an excess of the pure hormone labelled with a radioactive marker (see B and C), and subsequently separating the unreacted excess of pure hormone. The radioactivity remaining in the reaction-mixture is proportional to the amount of gamma globulin in excess of the amount required to react with the sample hormone. The concentration of the hormone is read by comparison of this reading against a standard curve.

E12 Answers

A. FALSE Cyclic AMP—stimulation is a common mechanism of peptide hormone action but steroid hormones penetrate the cell nucleus and activate gene transcription, thus stimulating the synthesis of specific proteins.

B. FALSE Hormones act as catalysts, without themselves being destroyed.

C. FALSE The main endocrine glands and tissues derived from the neural crest are the adrenal medulla, the parafollicular cells of the thyroid, endocrine cells of the alimentary tract, and the pancreatic islet cells.

D. TRUE Hormones are liberated into the blood stream.

E. TRUE In this respect also, hormones are catalysts.

5. METABOLISM

In measuring the size of a compartment of the body fluids by the dilution technique:-

A. the substance injected must be distributed evenly throughout the compartment
B. the amount (mass or weight) of substance injected must be known
C. the substance must be in physical solution in the compartment
D. the diffusion of substance into neighbouring compartments must be slow
E. the volume of sample taken from the compartment after equilibration must be accurately measured.

Answers overleaf

M1 Answers

A. TRUE   This must be so, otherwise the measured concentration, c, may not be representative of the whole compartment.

B. TRUE   The mass of substance injected must be known, even though it is usually expressed as the product a.V, when a is its concentration in the volume V injected.

C. FALSE   For example, Evans blue is adsorbed to the colloid particles of plasma albumin and therefore measures the albumin space without being in true solution.

D. TRUE   Rapid diffusion of the substance into other compartments results in a falsely low concentration in the final sample and a corresponding overestimate of the size of the space.

E. FALSE   The volume of the final sample is irrelevant, only the concentration, c, of the marker matters.

The plasma sodium ion concentration, $[Na^+]p$:-

A. is approximately the same as the intracellular sodium concentration, $[Na^+]c$
B. is exactly the same as the sodium concentration of the interstitial fluid, $[Na^+]i$
C. if low, is a reliable index of sodium depletion
D. is sometimes, despite normal sodium balance, influenced by the blood urea level.
E. is sometimes, despite normal sodium balance, influenced by low arterial oxygen tension.

Answers overleaf

M2 Answers

A. FALSE   The $[Na^+]c$ is very low, of the order of 5 mmol (mEq)/l. This vast gradient is maintained as a dynamic equilibrium by the 'sodium pump', a function of the cells whereby energy derived from aerobic metabolism and energy-rich phosphate bonds is used to force sodium ions out of the cells.

B. FALSE $[Na^+]p$ is approximately equal to $[Na^+]i$, but not exactly equal, although diffusion of electrolytes between the two spaces is free. The small difference is due to the fact that plasma protein, which behaves as an anion (positively charged), is non-diffusible. In such circumstances, the Donnan equilibrium predicts that the relation between *diffusible* ions is

$$\frac{[Na^+]p}{[Na^+]c} = \frac{[K^+]p}{[K^+]c} = \frac{[\text{any cation}^+]p}{[\text{any cation}^+]c} = \frac{[Cl^-]c}{[Cl^-]p} = \frac{[\text{any anion}^-]c}{[\text{any cation}^-]p}$$

C. FALSE   In sodium depletion, which in practice is always NaCl depletion, the losses are usually approximately isotonic (secretions from the gastrointestinal tract), and the extracellular space shrinks with $[Na]p$ remaining fairly constant until a late stage.

D. TRUE   In severe uraemia the high urea concentration in the plasma raises osmotic pressure and stimulates the hypothalamic osmoreceptors to retain water, resulting in the dilution of all electrolytes in the plasma.

E. TRUE   Cellular anoxia interferes with the sodium pump mechanism, resulting in a fall in $[Na^+]p$ and a rise in $[Na^+]c$.

The compound H_2A, where A is an unspecified atom or group of atoms, has a molecular weight X, and in aqueous solution dissociates practically completely according to the equation

$$H_2A \longrightarrow H^+ + HA^-.$$

It follows that:-

A. the anion HA^- is a base
B. the compound H_2A is a weak acid
C. a twice-normal (2N) aqueous solution of H_2A containing X grammes per litre
D. an aqueous solution of H_2A containing X grammes per litre is a twice osmolar solution
E. A could be HCO_3, i.e. H_2A could be carbonic acid, H_2CO_3, without contradicting the statements in the stem.

Answers overleaf

193

M3 Answers

A. TRUE   The hydrogen atom, H, may lose its orbital electron of unit negative electric charge, leaving the nucleus, a single particle called a proton, with its unit positive charge, H^+. An acid is defined as a proton donor, so H_2A behaves as an acid in the forward reaction $H_2A \longrightarrow H^+ + HA$. A base is defined as a proton acceptor, so A behaves as a base in the reverse reaction $H^+ + HA^- \longrightarrow H_2A$.

B. FALSE   The *strength* of an electrolyte refers to its degree of dissociation into oppositely charged ions (positive cations, negative anions) when dissolved in a suitable medium, usually water. A strong electrolyte dissociates practically completely, a weak electrolyte only to a slight extent. Therefore H_2A is a *strong* acid.

C. TRUE   A *normal* solution of a substance contains, per litre, the equivalent weight of the substance expressed in grammes. The equivalent weight of a substance is that weight of it which directly or indirectly reacts with one part by weight of hydrogen. From the equation $H_2A \longrightarrow 2H^+ + A^-$, it is clear that the molecule of H_2A has reacted with two atoms of hydrogen and so its equivalent weight is half its molecular weight. Therefore the *molar* solution specified contains 2 gramme-equivalents per litre.

D. TRUE   The osmotic pressure of a solution depends only on the number of particles of solute present and not at all on their nature. A solution containing the gramme-particle weight of any solute in 1 litre is defined as *osmolar*. When the gramme-molecular weight of H_2A is dissolved in 1 litre, each particle dissociates into *two* particles so the resultant solution is *twice* osmolar.

E. TRUE   Carbonic acid, H_2CO_3, *is* a strong acid: only about 1 part per thousand remains as H_2CO_3 molecules in aqueous solution, the rest form $H^+ + HCO_3$. The student may be confused by this: he knows that HCO_3^-, the bicarbonate ion, is an important element in the body buffering systems, and that a chemical buffer is defined as the mixture of a *weak* acid with its salt. The explanation lies in the fact that HCO_3^- is a physiological, not a chemical buffer. It owes its buffering effect to the fact that the reactions $HCO_3 + H^+ \longrightarrow H_2CO_3 \longrightarrow CO_2 + H_2O$ are greatly accelerated by the removal of CO_2 from the system by the lungs, or reversed by a reduction in pulmonary elimination of CO_2.

In a sample of arterial blood, the plasma bicarbonate concentration, $[HCO_3]p$,:-

A. is the same as the bicarbonate concentration in the red cells, $[HCO_3]c$
B. may be calculated by measuring the pH of the sample
C. depends partly upon alveolar ventilation
D. if measured after the blood has been equilibrated with a CO_2—nitrogen mixture of which the CO_2 has a partial pressure of 40 mm Hg, is called the plasma standard bicarbonate
E. if greater than 25 mmol/l (mEq/l), indicates metabolic alkalosis.

Answers overleaf

M4 Answers

A. FALSE   In the red cells, the protein (i.e. haemoglobin) concentration is far greater than in the plasma and is indiffusible: the diffusible electrolytes in the two compartments are therefore distributed according to the Donnan equilibrium (see Page 196). The red cells are more acid than the plasma, so

$$\frac{[H^+]c}{[H^+]p} = \frac{[HCO_3^-]p}{[HCO_3^-]c} > 1$$

i.e. the red cell and plasma bicarbonate concentrations differ from each other.

B. FALSE   The carbonic acid, hydrogen ion, and bicarbonate ions in a solution are linked by the chemical equation $H_2CO_3 \longrightarrow H^+ + HCO_3^-$, whence the law of Mass Action gives us

$$\frac{[H^+] \times [HCO_3^-]}{[H_2CO_3]} = \text{constant (the equilibrium constant)}$$

The value of the constant is known, but it is necessary to know two of the concentrations before the third can be calculated. Thus $[HCO_3^-]$ cannot be calculated from pH without knowing $[H_2CO_3]$.

C. TRUE $[H_2CO_3]$ is proportional to the partial pressure of CO_2 in the arterial sample, Pa_{CO_2}, and the latter is fixed by pulmonary ventilation. Therefore, $[HCO_3^-]p$ does depend partly on pulmonary ventilation.

D. FALSE   The definition of standard bicarbonate, $[HCO_3^-]s$, is that it is the $[HCO_3^-]p$ of a blood sample of haemoglobin concentration 14 g/dl, fully saturated with oxygen, and with a P_{CO_2} of 40 mm Hg. Changes in haemoglobin concentration have a definite effect on $[HCO_3^-]p$; the state of reduction/oxidation of haemoglobin also has an effect. Neither of these factors has been standardised correctly in item D.

E. FALSE   A *standard bicarbonate* greater than 25 mmol/l (mEq/l) indicates a metabolic alkalosis: no prediction about the metabolic component of acid-base balance can be made from the actual plasma bicarbonate. For example, a raised plasma bicarbonate might be due to an excess of carbonic acid, and therefore to a raised Pa_{CO_2}—underventilation or respiratory acidosis.

With regard to the absorption of iron:-

A. a well-balanced diet contains many times more iron in non-absorbable form, than in absorbable forms

B. when the iron stores are replete, no more iron from the alimentary tract lumen enters the mucosal cells

C. absorption of iron only takes place in the duodenum

D. the amount of absorbable iron in a well-balanced diet is much greater than the amount excreted

E. absorption of iron ceases in achlorhydria.

Answers overleaf

M5 Answers

A. TRUE   A good average daily diet contains $175 - 350 \mu mol$ $(10 - 20$ mg) of iron but only about one-tenth of this is available for absorption.

B. FALSE   Even when the iron stores are replete, iron enters the intestinal mucosal cells but is trapped there by combination with apoferritin to form ferritin and subsequently discarded by desquamation of that cell.

C. FALSE   Absorption of iron is *greatest* in the duodenum but it can be absorbed throughout the intestines, the capacity for absorption decreasing with the distance beyond the duodenum.

D. FALSE   The amount of absorbable iron in a well-balanced diet (see A above) is about $17 - 35 \mu mol$ $(1 - 2$ mg) per day. An adult male excretes about $17 \mu mol$ (1 mg) per day, a menstruating female about $35 \mu mol$ (2 mg) per day, and a pregnant woman requires a total of $52 \mu mol$ (3 mg) per day. Thus all menstruating women are teetering on the brink of iron-deficiency, while pregnant women definitely need supplements of iron.

E. FALSE   Absorption of iron is facilitated by the presence of hydrochloric acid, but can occur in its absence

Megaloblastic anaemia produced by Vitamin B_{12} (cyanocobalamin) deficiency:-

A. may occur after partial gastrectomy

B. only occurs with gastric histamine-fast achlorhydria

C. always responds to oral therapy with Vitamin B_{12} plus intrinsic factor

D. responds to 'physiological' doses of folic acid, i.e. $0.1 - 0.5$ mg daily

E. can be shown by examination of the marrow to respond to appropriate B_{12} therapy within 24 hours.

Answers overleaf

A. TRUE This is a rare complication of partial gastrectomy, and probably due to difficulty in freeing B_{12} from its bound form in food because of the reduced amount of acid secreted by the gastric remnant.

B. FALSE Histamine-fast achlorhydria is always present in conjunction with the gastric atrophy and lack of intrinsic factor production which produce pernicious anaemia. However, other causes of malabsorption of Vitamin B_{12} exist (see C below) and in these there is no necessity for the patient to be achlorhydric.

C. FALSE Pernicious anaemia always responds to oral B_{12} plus intrinsic factor. However, B_{12} deficiency may also be due to competition from the fish tapeworm, diphyllobothrium latum, or from abnormal bacteria in the bowel lumen, in such conditions as the blind loop syndrome, diverticula etc.

D. FALSE Fortunately, *small* doses of folic acid do not improve the haematological picture. Larger doses (5 – 15 mg daily) do, and if megaloblastic anaemia due to folic acid deficiency is diagnosed and treated with large doses of folic acid, a concomitant B_{12} deficiency may continue unrelieved with consequent damage to the nervous system despite correction of the blood picture.

E. TRUE The marrow shows striking change within 24 hours, although the reticulocyte count does not reach a peak till about the fifth or sixth day and the haemoglobin concentration then starts to rise.

A patient who has lost hydrochloric acid through vomiting due to pyloric obstruction is likely to have low:-

A. plasma chloride concentration
B. plasma potassium concentration
C. plasma urea concentration
D. plasma standard bicarbonate concentration
E. arterial carbon dioxide pressure (Pa_{CO_2}).

Answers overleaf

A. TRUE The loss of hydrogen and chloride ions in the acid vomitus results in a hypochloraemic metabolic alkalosis in the body fluids: at a given arterial carbon dioxide tension the plasma bicarbonate $[HCO_3^-]p$ is high and the plasma chloride $[Cl^-]p$ correspondingly low.

B. TRUE If the obstruction has caused persistent vomiting for more than 3 days, the patient is likely to be hypokalaemic—partly because of some potassium loss in the vomitus (at about 18 mmol/l), but mostly because of lack of dietary intake combined with inevitable continuing losses in the urine at about 40 mmol/l.

C. FALSE The extracellular depletion results in a reduction in urinary output and hence a rise in plasma urea concentration.

D. FALSE As indicated in A above, standard bicarbonate concentration rises—this is the definition of metabolic alkalosis.

E. TRUE The tendency towards alkalinity in the body fluids affects the respiratory centre via the chemoreceptors, causing respiratory depression and a respiratory acidosis that partially counteracts the metabolic alkalosis.

6. NEUROLOGY

Acute transection of the spinal cord at the 6th thoracic segment of the cord results in:-

A. anaesthesia below, normal sensation above, the level of the umbilicus
B. an increase in tone in the muscles of the lower limb, developing within one hour
C. bilateral positive (extensor, Babinski) plantar response
D. long term (at least for one month) systemic arterial hypotension
E. immediate incontinence of urine.

Conduction of a nervous impulse along an axon:-

A. needs no expenditure of energy
B. can only occur in one direction in a particular neuron
C. is more rapid in small fibres than in large
D. is more rapid in myelinated than in non-myelinated fibres
E. is more sensitive to anoxia than is synaptic transmission.

Answers overleaf

N1 Answers

A. FALSE   The dermatome at the level of the umbilicus is T10, so that in this case the upper limit of the anaesthesia extends well above the umbilicus.

B. FALSE   The period of 'spinal shock' lasts several weeks in man; during this time there is a total loss of all function, including reflex activity, distal to the block. Increased tone does not develop till this period has passed.

C. TRUE   The Babinski response is characteristic of interruption of the pyramidal pathways.

D. FALSE   The sixth thoracic segment is below the level of the sympathetic outflow and so hypotension due to loss of sympathetic vasoconstrictor activity will not occur.

E. FALSE   During the period of spinal shock the bladder is atonic and no urine is passed unless the bladder is allowed to overfill, when retention with overflow-incontinence may occur.

N2 Answers

A. FALSE   The transmission of a nervous impulse along an axon is an electrochemical process involving movements of ions between the intra- and extracellular compartments and changes in electrical potential across the cell membrane.

B. FALSE   Neuronal transmission proceeds equally well in either direction.

C. FALSE   Transmission is more rapid in large fibres than in small.

D. TRUE   This is mostly due to the insulating properties of the myelin sheath, but also partly to the lower electrical resistance of the thicker axon.

E. FALSE   Synaptic transmission is much more sensitive to anoxia than is neuronal.

Transmission of a nerve impulse across a synapse:-

A. can only occur in one direction
B. involves the release of a transmitter substance at the pre-synaptic terminals
C. can take place despite the release of an inhibitory transmitter substance at the pre-synaptic terminals
D. depends on local depolarization in the membrane of the post-synaptic cell
E. is more rapid in circuits containing several synapses than in long fibre tracts.

With regard to the stretch (myotactic) reflex:-

A. it is the *only* monosynaptic reflex in the human
B. the afferent arc originates in the Golgi tendon organ
C. the efferent arc starts in the α – motor neuron
D. the annulospiral receptor is relaxed when the muscle contracts
E. stimulation of the afferent arc may produce inhibition of contraction of the antagonistic muscles.

Answers overleaf

N3 Answers

A. TRUE In this respect synaptic transmission differs sharply from neuronal conduction.

B. TRUE The knob at the pre-synaptic terminal releases a specific chemical transmitter that diffuses across the gap to the post-synaptic cell.

C. TRUE At the same synapse there may be pre-synaptic knobs releasing an inhibitory transmitter as well as knobs releasing the excitatory transmitter. The net effect on the post-synaptic cell is the algebraic sum of the inhibitory and excitatory effects.

D. TRUE If the algebraic sum of the inhibitory and excitatory transmitters achieves a high enough excitatory post-synaptic potential due to depolarization, the post-synaptic cell fires a propagated spike action potential.

E. FALSE Each synapse involves a delay of about half a millisecond.

N4 Answers

A. TRUE All other reflexes involve more than one synapse.

B. FALSE The Golgi tendon organs are activated by contraction of the muscle, their discharge relays via an internuncial synapse in the cord to the α-motor neuron, and the latter produces inhibition of muscle contraction and protection of the muscle from excessive contraction.

C. TRUE

D. TRUE The annulospiral receptor is wound round the central, non-contractile part of the intrafusal fibre. Since the latter is not attached to the points of origin and insertion of the muscle, it does not contract when the muscle shortens but is relaxed.

E. TRUE Some collaterals of the afferent fibre may innervate inhibitory internuncial neurones and these in turn inhibit the activity of α-motor neurones supplying antagonistic muscles—'reciprocal inhibition'.

Cerebral blood flow:-

A. is independent of changes in mean arterial blood pressure in the range 75 – 125 mm Hg
B. increases with raised arterial carbon dioxide tension
C. falls with a lowered arterial oxygen tension in the range 30 – 50 mm Hg
D. falls immediately with a small rise in intracranial pressure
E. is sensitive to small changes in the viscosity of the blood.

The cerebrospinal fluid:-

A. volume in the spinal subarachnoid space is much greater than the volume within the skull
B. is formed mostly by the choroid plexuses of the ventricles
C. is formed at a greater rate if cerebral oxygen consumption is increased
D. has a volume between 1 and 1½ litres in the adult
E. in different anatomical sites varies in the concentrations of its constituents.

Answers overleaf

N5 Answers

A. TRUE   This is the process known as *autoregulation*: it seems to be mediated by dilatation of small intracranial arteries, and cerebral blood flow remains constant as arterial pressure falls until the latter is less than 50 mm Hg.

B. TRUE   An increase in carbon dioxide tension is the most powerful stimulus to changes in cerebral blood flow.

C. FALSE   While cerebral blood flow remains constant over a wide range of arterial oxygen tension, a fall in the latter below 50 mm Hg results in an *increase* in cerebral blood flow due to vasodilatation of intracranial arteries.

D. FALSE   In the early phases of rising intracranial pressure, cerebral blood flow remains constant: it is only when the pressure-differential between arterial blood pressure and intracerebral pressure falls below 40 mm Hg that the cerebral blood flow falls.

E. FALSE   Moderate changes in the viscosity of the circulating blood have little effect on cerebral blood flow.

N6 Answers

A. TRUE   The volume in the spine is about 75 ml, that within the skull 55 ml.

B. TRUE

C. TRUE   The formation of cerebrospinal fluid (CSF) is directly related to cerebral oxygen consumption.

D. FALSE   The volume is about 150 ml (see the answer to A above).

E. TRUE   The concentrations of dissolved solutes are altered in certain places, viz. the ventricles and the spinal subarachnoid space, by diffusion of water across the lining walls.

Factors tending to increase intracranial pressure include:-

A. hypercapnia (raised carbon dioxide tension)
B. hypoxia (lowered oxygen tension)
C. hypothermia
D. systemic arterial hypotension (in circumstances where the brain is undamaged)
E. strangling.

Passage of a nerve impulse:-

A. along an axon is facilitated by hypothermia
B. occurs at a steady rate throughout the length of the axon
C. along large, heavily myelinated nerve fibres occurs at speeds approaching that of an electric current
D. across all synapses outside the central nervous system is effected by the chemical transmitter, acetylcholine
E. across all synapses within the central nervous system is never effected by acetylcholine.

Answers overleaf

N7 Answers

A. TRUE   The vasodilator effect of hypercapnia acting on the cerebral arterioles increases the cerebral blood volume. The mechanisms include a local direct effect and a remote action via the chemoreceptors in the great vessels.

B. TRUE   Hypoxia, like hypercapnia, produces vasodilatation by the same two mechanisms.

C. FALSE   Hypothermia results in vasoconstriction and thus lowers the cerebral blood volume and so the intracranial pressure.

D. FALSE   In the absence of brain damage, the phenomenon of auto-regulation keeps the cerebral blood flow constant despite a wide range of variation in systemic arterial blood pressure. However, in the severely damaged brain, autoregulation is lost.

E. TRUE   A constricting agent applied around the neck obstructs the veins, with their blood at low pressure, more completely than the high-pressure arteries. The consequent damming back of the cerebral venous blood raises the volume of the intracranial blood and hence increases intracranial tension.

N8 Answers

A. FALSE   Hypothermia slows down the rate of passage of the nervous impulse.

B. FALSE   In myelinated fibres, the impulse 'jumps' rapidly from one node of Ranvier to the next—the so-called *saltatory* conduction.

C. FALSE   Conduction is certainly more rapid in thick, heavily myelinated nerve fibres than in other nerves, but only reaches at most 100 m/sec. An electric current travels about 100 km in 10 msec.

D. FALSE   Acetylcholine is the chemical transmitter liberated at all peripheral nerve endings *except* postganglionic sympathetic fibres, where adrenaline is the transmitter. It is also now becoming clear that vasoactive intestinal polypeptide (VIP) is the transmitter at many synapses with endocrine glands of the alimentary tract.

E. FALSE   Information about chemical transmitters at synapses within the central nervous system is incomplete, but it is clear that acetylcholine is the transmitter at least at some: for example, certain cells in the cerebral cortex and in the pyramidal system, and the Renshaw cells of the anterior horn that inhibit antagonists when muscle spindles are stimulated.

Factors involved in the onset of fatigue in voluntary muscle include:-

A. failure of conduction in the motor nerve
B. failure of the transmission of the nerve impulse across the synapse to the motor end plate
C. failure to initiate action potentials in the muscle
D. stimulation of gamma-efferent nerve fibres to the muscle spindles from higher centres in the extrapyramidal tracts
E. use of repeated electrical stimulation of the same muscle group, by comparison with the effect of natural activity.

Substances that block neuromuscular conduction by competing with transmitter acetylcholine at the motor end plate include:-

A. neomycin
B. thiopentone
C. halothane
D. neostigmine
E. botulinus toxin.

Answers overleaf

N9 Answers

A. B. & C. FALSE   All these aspects of neuromuscular activity remain unimpaired despite rapid repetitive contractions for a prolonged period. The major factor producing fatigue is biochemical: the accumulation of lactic acid due to anaerobic metabolism when the oxygen demands of the actively contracting muscle outstrip the available oxygen in the blood supply.

D. FALSE   There is no physiological evidence in favour of this mechanism to explain the higher centres being involved in muscle fatigue.

E. TRUE   During natural activity, fatigue in any one group of muscles is postponed by neighbouring groups with similar functions taking over the activity. This spreading of the load cannot happen when artificial stimulation of an electric current is used.

N10 Answers

A. TRUE   Although neomycin blocks the release of transmitter acetylcholine at the pre-synaptic terminals (see answer to N. 14, E), it also acts as a competitive antagonist at the motor end plate.

B. TRUE   Thus thiopentone used for induction of anaesthesia potentiates the effect of any subsequently administered relaxant drug.

C. TRUE

D. FALSE   Neostigmine is an anticholinesterase, and its effects on neuromuscular condition are due to that property.

E. FALSE   Botulinus toxin blocks neuromuscular conduction by interfering with the release of acetylcholine from the presynaptic terminals.

Interference with transmission at somatic neuromuscular junctions may be due to:-

A. thiamine deficiency
B. carcinoma of the bronchus
C. diabetes mellitus
D. hyperthyroidism
E. hypothyroidism

When the continuity of a nerve fibre is interrupted, the distal segment:-

A. completely loses its excitability within 12 hours
B. afferent fibres become inexcitable sooner than efferent (motor) fibres
C. changes are more rapid in infants than in adults
D. changes occur more rapidly if the tissues are warm rather than cold
E. shows, in the period before it becomes inexcitable, an increase in the amplitude of its action potential.

Answers overleaf

N11 Answers

A. B. C. D. & E. TRUE The functional disturbance is associated with structural changes, especially in the presynaptic terminals. A, C, D, and E are direct mechanisms: the way in which carcinoma of the bronchus (and, less often, other malignancies) produce their effect is unknown, but may involve an immunological mechanism since an anti-neuronal antibody has been identified in the serum of patients with carcinomatous neuropathies.

N12 Answers

A. FALSE Excitability does not completely disappear until, in most nerve fibres, about 72 hours have passed—in some of the largest diameter fibres it may take 5 days.

B. TRUE The speed with which degeneration occurs seems to be related to the diameter of the fibres, and the afferent fibres, smaller on average than the efferent, degenerate faster.

C. TRUE

D. TRUE Presumably this is related to the greater metabolic demands of warm tissues.

E. FALSE There is a general gradual reduction in excitability from the time of division of the nerve until it becomes completely inexcitable. Thus the threshold for excitability begins to rise, the conduction velocity gradually slows, and the amplitude of the action potential gradually falls.

When the nerve supplying a somatic muscle has been divided:-

A. the muscle becomes less sensitive to acetylcholine
B. a needle electrode placed within the muscle will, after the first two minutes, detect no electrical activity
C. the temperature of the overlying skin immediately falls
D. the electrical resistance of the overlying skin immediately falls
E. the strength-duration curve of the muscle 'shifts to the right', i.e., a larger than normal electrical current is required to produce a just visible contraction of the muscle when applied for a standard duration.

Following sympathetic denervation of the lower limb:-

A. resting tone in the skin blood vessels is permanently abolished
B. vasoconstriction of skin vessels in response to a fall in core temperature is permanently abolished
C. vasodilatatiqn in muscle vessels in response to exercise occurs normally
D. vasoconstriction in muscle vessels in response to a change in posture from supine to erect is permanently abolished
E. sweating is permanently abolished.

Answers overleaf

N13 Answers

A. FALSE   Not just the motor-end plate, but the whole muscle becomes very sensitive to acetylcholine.

B. FALSE   The phenomenon described in A above results in hyperexcitability of the denervated muscle which expresses itself in spontaneous 'fibrillation spike potentials'.

C. FALSE   When the nerve is cut its sympathetic fibres innervating the skin blood vessels are interrupted and the resultant release of vasomotor tone produces an increased blood flow, and hence an increased temperature, in the skin.

D. FALSE   The sudomotor fibres to the sweat glands have also been interrupted and the skin becomes dry, and therefore more resistant to the passage of an electric current.

E. TRUE   The presence of significant motor nerve injury can be diagnosed, and the progress of regeneration followed, by serial measurements plotting strength-duration curves.

N14 Answers

A. FALSE   Resting skin blood flow acutely increases about tenfold, but this effect gradually becomes less until the flow stabilizes, about 14 days after the sympathectomy, at about two-fold. The mechanism of the return of most of the tone probably includes an increased sensitivity to circulating catecholamines.

B. TRUE   Vascular reflexes mediated by the sympathetic are permanently abolished. This applies to the lower limb, but in the upper limb there may be some recovery of vascular reflexes—the mechanism is unknown.

C. TRUE   Vasodilatation in muscles during excercise is a local phenomenon, mediated by the direct effect of metabolites and local nervous reflexes.

D. TRUE   This is another example of abolition of a vascular reflex mediated by the sympathetic—as in B above.

E. TRUE   Hence the value of sympathectomy in patients suffering with hyperhidrosis.

7. UROLOGY

With respect to renal tubular function:-

A. sodium is mainly reabsorbed in the proximal tubule
B. potassium is mainly reabsorbed in the distal tubule
C. ammonia is excreted into the proximal tubule
D. hydrogen ions are excreted into the distal tubule
E. four-fifths of water reabsorption occurs in the proximal tubule.

In an adult on a normal intake of food and water, 24-hourly urinary outputs compatible with normal health include:-

A. water, 0.5 litre
B. sodium, 20 mmol (meq)
C. potassium, 80 mmol (meq)
D. protein, 500 mg
E. total titratable acid, 200 mmol (meq).

Answers overleaf

U1 Answers

A. TRUE

B. & C. FALSE   The main site is the proximal tubule.

C. D. & E. TRUE

U2 Answers

  A. FALSE   The normal range of urine volume on a normal diet is 1 – 2 litres. The reader may have marked this question as true because a subject can maintain normal health in the face of a reduced water intake if his daily urinary excretion remains as high as 500 ml, but if he only passes this quantity despite a *normal* water intake, something is wrong.

  B. FALSE   The sodium intake in a normal diet is at least 75 mmol (meq), and so an amount of this order should be passed in the urine.

  C. TRUE

  D. FALSE   The glomerular filter does permit the passage of a small quantity of protein, but the upper limit of concentration in the urine of a healthy subject is 150 mg/litre so the upper limit for the normal output is about 300 mg.

  E. TRUE   The total acid load (other than carbonic acid) resulting from diet and metabolism is of the order of 100 – 200 mmol (meq) daily.

With respect to renal clearance values and the expression $\frac{UV}{P}$:-

A. U always refers to the urinary urea concentration
B. P refers to plasma volume
C. creatinine clearance depends on the rate of urine flow
D. creatinine clearance measures effective renal plasma flow
E. clearance is usually expressed as a volume per unit time, e.g. ml/min.

U4 Questions

With reference to the normal control of micturition:-

A. during the filling of the bladder with 500 ml of liquid, the change in *intrinsic* bladder pressure is less than 10 cm of water
B. during the filling of the bladder with 500 ml of liquid, the change in *overall* pressure within the bladder is mostly due to increased intra-abdominal pressure
C. when the subject is asked to stop micturition after he has started the act, the mechanism brought into action is the 'internal sphincter' at the bladder neck
D. the 'external' or distal posterior urethral sphincter is composed exclusively of striated muscle
E. the striated muscle of the external sphincter is responsible for continence during sleep.

Answers overleaf

U3 Answers

A. FALSE U refers to the urinary concentration of the substance of which the clearance is being measured. Thus, only when *urea* clearance is being measured does U refer to urinary urea concentration.

B. FALSE P refers to the concentration in the plasma of the substance whose clearance is being measured.

C. FALSE Unlike urea, whose clearance varies with the rate of urine flow, creatinine gives stable clearance values over a wide range of urinary excretion rate.

D. FALSE Most of the endogenous creatinine in the urine gets there via glomerular filtration, only a little by tubular excretion; thus creatinine clearance represents glomerular filtration rate rather than total effective renal plasma flow.

E. TRUE *Clearance* of a substance is the volume of plasma cleared of that substance in unit time by means of excretion in the urine.

U4 Answers

A. TRUE Intrinsic bladder pressure is calculated by subtracting intra-abdominal (e.g. rectal) pressure from the total intravesical pressure: in the normal subject, intrinsic bladder pressure rises hardly at all during filling of the bladder.

B. TRUE Total bladder pressure does rise, almost entirely due to an increase in intra-abdominal pressure.

C. FALSE The mechanism involved in stopping micturition is the external sphincter.

D. FALSE The external sphincter has two components: an 'extrinsic', consisting of striated muscle, that by voluntary contraction stops micturition and an 'intrinsic' of unstriated muscle that then empties the urine in the posterior urethra back into the bladder.

E. FALSE The external sphincter striated muscle is relaxed during sleep.

Urine with a markedly acid reaction (pH < 5.0):-

A. contains bicarbonate ions in greater than average concentration
B. is within normal limits
C. contains ammonium ions in greater than average concentration
D. probably contains little or no sodium
E. contains more $H_2PO_4^-$ than $HPO_4^=$.

Answers overleaf

U5 Answers

A. FALSE The more acid a solution, the more bicarbonate (HCO_3^-) ions become displaced from the solution through the formation of CO_2 gas (evolved) and water. Thus

$$H^+ + HCO_3^- \longrightarrow H_2CO_3 \longrightarrow H_2O + CO_2$$

The quantitative relationship is expressed by the Henderson-Hasselbalch equation

$$pH = pK + \log_{10} \frac{[HCO_3]}{P_{CO_2}}$$

The pK and P_{CO_2} of urine are approximately the same as plasma, so if the pH of the urine is 5

$$5 = 6.1 + \log_{10} [HCO_3] - \log_{10} 1.2$$

$$\text{or } \log_{10} [HCO_3] = -1.1 + \log_{10} 1.2 = \bar{1}.989$$

$$\text{or } [HCO_3] = 1 \text{ mmol/l}$$

B. TRUE A normal diet contains sulphur, phosphorus and similar non-metals that form non-volatile acids that must be excreted in the urine. The average daily load of such acids, about 200 mmol, ensures that some samples of normal urine are strongly acidic.

C. TRUE The ammonium ions (NH_4^+) derived from ammonia (NH_3) produced in the liver help to balance the excess anions (phosphate, sulphate) in acid urine.

D. TRUE Sodium ions are retained in the body to help in balancing the excess anions in the body fluids. Ammonium cannot be employed for this purpose as high concentrations are toxic.

E. TRUE The tendency to a high concentration of hydrogen ions titrates the dihydrogen to the monohydrogen phosphate form—

$$H^+ + HPO_4^= \longrightarrow H_2PO_4^-$$

Factors increasing glomerular filtration rate include:-

A. increased plasma colloid osmotic pressure
B. constriction of the glomerular afferent arterioles
C. dilatation of the glomerular efferent arterioles
D. respiratory alkalosis
E. saline-depletion.

Blood urea concentration:-

A. in health is usually in the range 20 – 30 mg/dl (3.5 – 5 mmol/l)
B. does not rise after a protein-rich meal
C. below the normal range, e.g. 12 mg/dl (2 mmol/l) signifies that the kidneys are working particularly well
D. falls in a patient bleeding profusely from a duodenal ulcer
E. is usually above the normal range on the first morning after a major surgical operation.

Answers overleaf

U6 Answers

A. FALSE The plasma colloid osmotic pressure opposes the filtration-force of the hydrostatic pressure within the glomerulus, so that an increased colloid osmotic pressure reduces the glomerular filtration rate.

B. & C. FALSE Constriction of the afferent arterioles and dilatation of the efferent arterioles both tend to reduce the hydrostatic pressure within the glomerulus and hence the filtration-force.

D. FALSE Respiratory alkalosis, i.e. a hyperventilation-induced washing of carbon dioxide out of the blood, results in a widespread vasoconstriction and a fall in cardiac output as a whole, and in renal perfusion in particular.

E. FALSE Saline-depletion results in a contraction of the extracellular space, and hence of the plasma (which is a part of the extracellular space) and hence of the blood volume. Again cardiac output falls, and so does renal perfusion and thus glomerular filtration rate is likely to fall too.

U7 Answers

A. TRUE

B. FALSE A moderate rise to about 7 mmol/l commonly occurs during the first four hours after a protein-rich meal, particularly if there is no diuresis.

C. FALSE A low blood urea concentration signifies that the rate of production of urea (in the liver) is abnormally low and thus indicates hepatic dysfunction rather than super-healthy kidneys!

D. FALSE Blood in the bowel constitutes a massive protein meal, and severe bleeding results in diminished renal perfusion, a lowered glomerular filtration rate, and oliguria or anuria. Both these effects tend to raise blood urea concentration.

E. TRUE The factors responsible include (1) limitation of intake of water during and shortly after surgery and anaesthesia; (2) inevitable oliguria due to increased output of ADH (pure water retention) and aldosterone (sodium-linked water retention) in response to trauma; (3) increased catabolism and therefore increased production of urea in response to trauma; and possibly (4) inadequate restitution of blood, plasma or saline loss resulting from the surgical procedure.

III. PATHOLOGY

1. INFLAMMATION AND REPAIR

Multinucleate giant cells are seen in man in association with:-

A. cat-scratch disease
B. measles
C. rheumatic fever
D. syphilis
E. tuberculosis.

Macrophages:-

A. are derived from blood monocytes
B. can multiply
C. fuse to form multinucleate giant cells
D. live longer than neutrophils
E. produce immunoglobulins.

Answers overleaf

Infl. 1 Answers

A. TRUE Occasional giant cells are to be seen in the zone of macrophages which surrounds the central necrotic area.

B. TRUE Typical giant cells occur: they were first and independently described in 1931 by two pathologists, Warthin in America and Finkeldey in Germany. These giant cells are very large with many close-packed nuclei throughout the cytoplasm. They are most dramatically observed in the lymphoid tissue of tonsils or appendices excised in the prodromal stage of infection before the characteristic skin rash develops.

C. TRUE The basic cardiac lesion of rheumatic fever is the Aschoff body. This is situated in the interstitial tissue of the myocardium close to a coronary arteriole. It is fusiform with a central necrotic area and surrounding pleomorphic cellular exudate. The predominant cell resembles a macrophage and multinucleate forms often occur—the Aschoff giant cell. Ludwig Aschoff (1866 – 1942), German pathologist, was one of the great pathologists of all time.

D. TRUE Occasional giant cells are seen in the gumma—the typical lesion of tertiary syphilis.

E. TRUE

Infl. 2 Answers

A. TRUE Most macrophages are derived from migrating blood monocytes, which are produced in the bone marrow.

B. TRUE Many macrophages are destroyed, but some undergo division to form small round cells, which in turn mature to macrophages.

C. TRUE Current evidence indicates that multinucleate giant cells seen in inflammatory processes and as a reaction to foreign material form by fusion of mononuclear precursor cells —macrophages. Repeated nuclear division of macrophages without cytoplasmic separation probably does not occur.

D. TRUE Neutrophils have a short life span of only three to four days outside the blood stream. Migrated monocytes live longer, but their life span is very variable: some live only a few weeks before death; others persist for much longer, especially if they have ingested insoluble material; and yet others multiply.

E. FALSE Although the presence of macrophages often appears to enhance the immune response, the actual production of antibodies occurs in plasma cells.

Neutrophil granulocytes:-

A. antagonise the action of histamine
B. are actively phagocytic
C. are found in pus
D. can be killed by bacterial products
E. contain lysosomes.

Tissue eosinophilia is a characteristic of:-

A. amoebiasis
B. bronchial asthma
C. filariasis
D. tertiary syphilis
E. viral infections.

Answers overleaf

Infl. 3 Answers

A. FALSE   The granules of eosinophils however contain an antihistamine substance.

B. TRUE   A major function of neutrophils is to phagocytose and destroy micro-organisms.

C. TRUE   Many virulent micro-organisms are pyogenic; they cause acute inflammation with abundant neutrophil emigration and local toxic damage producing tissue necrosis. Enzymes from the neutrophils help in digesting dead tissue. Pus is rich in neutrophils ('pus cells'), both living and dead, together with bacteria and products of tissue breakdown.

D. TRUE   Neutrophils are able to destroy many micro-organisms; however, some bacteria produce potent toxins which are able to destroy neutrophils. Such toxins—leucocidins—are produced by both *staphylococcus pyogenes* and *streptococcus pyogenes*.

E. TRUE   Neutrophil lysosomes contain a rich variety of enzymes that can digest most biological materials when liberated from the cell or into the cell's phagocytic vacuoles.

Infl. 4 Answers

A. FALSE   Relatively little cellular reaction occurs in amoebic lesions unless there is superimposed secondary infection. Even in the so-called 'amoebic abscess' only scanty neutrophils are present.

B. TRUE   In the acute attack eosinophil infiltration of the bronchial mucosa is an important feature.

C. TRUE   Tissue eosinophilia is a feature of infestation by many varieties of worms.

D. FALSE   The lesions in tertiary syphilis are characterised by tissue destruction and an infiltrate of lymphocytes, plasma cells and macrophages. These features are typically seen in the syphilitic gumma.

E. FALSE   In the very early stage of virus infections there may be a neutrophil cellular reaction, but the more general reaction is lymphocytic.

Healing of a fracture is delayed by:-

A. deficiency of calcium
B. deficiency of protein
C. deficiency of vitamin C
D. deficiency of vitamin D
E. immobilisation.

Necrosis is an important feature of the lesions in:-

A. acute anterior poliomyelitis
B. lobar pneumonia
C. rheumatic fever
D. tertiary syphilis
E. viral hepatitis.

Answers overleaf

Infl. 5 Answers

A. B. C. & D. TRUE   All these factors are essential for new bone formation. Vitamin C deficiency impairs both collagen synthesis and bone production. With lack of vitamin D or of calcium abundant callus may form, but it will fail to calcify. Protein—and especially the sulphur-containing aminoacids—are essential for the formation of collagen and bone matrix.

E. FALSE   Movement of any significant degree is harmful. Reparative granulation tissue is damaged causing haemorrhage and an inflammatory reaction.

Infl. 6 Answers

A. TRUE   The basic lesion is necrosis of anterior horn cells in the spinal cord and of cranial nerve cells in the cerebral medulla in the bulbar form. The corresponding axons degenerate and the changes are irreversible.

B. FALSE   Destruction of lung tissue does not normally occur. The acute inflammatory exudate within the alveoli usually undergoes resolution with no residual damage.

C. TRUE   The classical microscopic Aschoff node (see also Question Infl. 1. C) has a small central necrotic focus. In addition, the characteristic subcutaneous rheumatic nodule consists of an area of fibrinoid necrosis surrounded by a granulomatous reaction.

D. TRUE   The typical lesion is the gumma, which consists of a large necrotic central zone surrounded by chronic inflammatory cells including occasional multinucleate giant cells.

E. TRUE   In all forms of viral hepatitis there is necrosis of single cells or groups of cells in the liver lobule. In severe infections, especially with Type B viral hepatitis (homologous serum jaundice), there may be massive liver cell necrosis and death from liver failure.

Caseation commonly occurs in:-

A. actinomycosis
B. gas gangrene
C. sarcoidosis
D. staphylococcal infections
E. tuberculosis.

Monocytes are:-

A. actively motile
B. actively phagocytic
C. able to transform into lymphocytes
D. the typical cell of early acute inflammation
E. the typical cell of infectious mononucleosis (glandular fever).

Answers overleaf

233

Infl. 7 Answers

A. B. C. & D. FALSE   Necrosis occurs in all these conditions though in sarcoidosis it is minimal. However, the peculiar form of necrosis known as caseation does not occur in these conditions.

E. TRUE   Caseation has a firm cheese-like gross appearance: histologically it appears as granular amorphous eosinophilic material with no indication of former tissue architecture. It is particularly associated with tuberculous infection, but an essentially similar appearance can occur in syphilitic gummas and in some infarcts and necrotic tumours. In the usual type of coagulative necrosis ghost tissue structure is present for a long time.

Infl. 8 Answers

A. TRUE   Monocytes, like neutrophils, are actively motile. Their passage through the wall of venules in an inflamed area is an active process; they wander through tissue spaces and their movements appear to be mediated by chemotaxis.

B. TRUE   The phagocytic property of blood monocytes can be used to label them with ingested carbon particles in their cytoplasm. The labelled cells can then be observed to pass through blood vessel walls and into tissue spaces where they transform to very actively phagocytic macrophages.

C. FALSE   At certain stages of their life lymphocytes and monocytes can look very much alike. However, they are distinct cell types and transformation between them does not occur.

D. FALSE   In the early stages of acute inflammation neutrophils are the dominant cell. Later monocytes appear in increasing numbers and their numbers may then be further boosted by multiplication of the emigrated cells (neutrophils are not capable of further multiplication).

E. FALSE   Although the abnormal blood cells somewhat resemble monocytes they are T lymphoblasts.

Bacterial infections characterised by an intense emigration of neutrophils include:-

A. *Escherichia coli*
B. *Mycobacterium tuberculosis*
C. *Neisseria gonorrhoeae*
D. *Salmonella typhi*
E. *Streptococcus pneumoniae.*

Answers overleaf

Infl. 9 Answers

A. TRUE The two major causes of pyogenic infection in man are *Staphylococcus pyogenes* and *Streptococcus pyogenes*, but there are other common pyogenic bacteria. *Esch. coli* is associated with pyogenic infections in the abdomen (appendicitis, diverticulitis, peritonitis) and in many other parts of the body (urinary tract infections, wound infections).

B. FALSE Early in a tuberculous infection there may be a mild neutrophil response, but the main cellular response is by lymphocytes, plasma cells and macrophages.

C. TRUE Its close relative the meningococcus (*Neisseria meningitidis*) also produces a suppurative reaction.

D. FALSE The inflammatory cellular reaction is mainly of macrophages, lymphocytes and plasma cells. Neutrophils only appear in significant numbers in secondarily infected ulcerated lesions.

E. TRUE The alveolar exudate in lobar pneumonia consists predominantly of neutrophils.

2. TUMOURS

Adenocarcinoma is the commonest type of primary malignant epithelial tumour to occur in the:-

A. colon
B. lung
C. oesophagus
D. stomach
E. uterine cervix.

Squamous cell carcinoma is the usual type of primary malignant epithelial tumour arising in the:-

A. bladder
B. prostate
C. rectum
D. skin
E. tongue.

Answers overleaf

Tum. 1 Answers

A. TRUE Other types of carcinoma are rarely seen.

B. FALSE Various types of carcinoma arise here including adenocarcinomas, oat cell carcinomas, alveolar cell carcinomas and anaplastic carcinomas, but the commonest type is squamous cell carcinoma.

C. FALSE Occasional adenocarcinomas arise from mucous glands or from ectopic or metaplastic gastric mucosa, but the vast majority of carcinomas are of squamous cell type.

D. TRUE Other types of carcinoma are rare.

E. FALSE Only about five per cent of cervical carcinomas are adenocarcinomas; the rest are of squamous cell type.

Tum. 2 Answers

A. FALSE Most malignant bladder tumours are transitional cell carcinomas, though they may show foci of squamous metaplasia. Pure squamous cell carcinomas account for only 2 – 3 per cent of bladder tumours and adenocarcinomas are even less common.

B. FALSE Prostatic carcinomas are nearly all adenocarcinomas.

C. FALSE Nearly all rectal carcinomas are adenocarcinomas, but a few squamous cell carcinomas occur at the ano-rectal margin.

D. TRUE The two common carcinomas of the skin are the basal cell and squamous cell types. Malignant melanomas are much less common.

E. TRUE Apart from an occasional carcinoma of glandular origin, the vast majority arise from surface epithelium and are of squamous cell type.

238

Features that are more characteristic of benign tumours than malignant tumours include:-

A. anaplasia
B. capsule formation
C. infiltration of surrounding tissue
D. many mitotic figures
E. slow rate of growth.

Metastases in lymph nodes are a common feature of:-

A. basal cell carcinoma
B. fibroadenoma
C. malignant melanoma
D. seminoma
E. squamous cell carcinoma.

Blood borne metastases are a common feature of:-

A. astrocytoma
B. basal cell carcinoma
C. osteosarcoma
D. prostatic carcinoma
E. squamous cell carcinoma of the tongue.

Answers overleaf

Tum. 3 Answers

A. FALSE   Benign tumours are well-differentiated and closely resemble their tissue of origin.

B. TRUE   This is a typical feature of benign tumours and is much less often seen in malignant tumours.

C. FALSE   Invasion of adjacent tissues is the major feature of malignant tumours.

D. & E. FALSE and TRUE   The vast majority of malignant tumours grow more rapidly than benign ones and the mitotic rate is a rough measure of the rate of growth.

Tum. 4 Answers

A. FALSE   These tumours are malignant and spread locally but very rarely produce metastases.

B. FALSE   This is a benign tumour.

C. D. & E. TRUE   In all these tumours lymphatic spread is common and important.

Tum. 5 Answers

A. FALSE   These tumours invade locally. They do not spread by lymphatics or blood but may seed within the cerebral ventricles and subarachnoid space.

B. FALSE   These tumours are locally invasive. Rarely, lymphatic spread has been recorded: blood spread is an extreme rarity.

C. TRUE   Blood spread is, unfortunately, very common, especially to the lungs.

D. TRUE   Again, blood spread is important. Sites of metastasis include the bones in which osteoplastic deposits with new bone formation are quite common.

E. FALSE   Distant spread is almost entirely by the lymphatic route.

Agents causing cancer in man include:-

A. arsenic
B. asbestos
C. ionising radiation
D. thorotrast
E. ultra-violet light.

An increased incidence of cancer occurs in:-

A. aniline dye workers
B. bus conductors
C. chimney sweeps
D. shale-oil workers
E. wood workers.

Answers overleaf

Tum. 6 Answers

A. TRUE Workers using arsenic and patients with a prolonged intake of medicines containing inorganic arsenicals are prone to develop skin cancer. Occupational exposure to arsenic is also associated with an enhanced incidence of lung cancer.

B. TRUE There is a definite association between exposure to asbestos and the development of lung cancer and of pleural mesothelioma.

C. TRUE Several types of tumour are associated with exposure to ionising radiation: they include carcinomas of the skin and thyroid, and also leukaemia (see also question Gen. 3).

D. TRUE Thorotrast was used quite extensively as a contrast medium in angiography from 1930 to 1953. It was administered parenterally and removed from the circulation by phagocytic reticulo-endothelial cells and stored by them in the liver, spleen and bone marrow. After a long latent period—a mean of over 20 years—tumours have developed in the liver (angiosarcoma and hepatoma) and in bones (osteosarcoma).

E. TRUE Prolonged exposure to sunlight, especially in fair-skinned people, leads to an increased incidence of squamous cell and basal cell carcinomas, and of malignant melanomas.

Tum. 7 Answers

A. TRUE Exposure to aniline and related aromatic amines (e.g. alpha- and beta-naphthylamine and benzidine) used in dyeing and in the manufacture of rubber, plastics and insulated cables is associated with the development of bladder cancer.

B. FALSE They have no special prevalence of cancer.

C. TRUE This was the first documented occupational cancer—scrotal cancer due to soot. The association was described in 1775 by Percivall Pott (1814 – 88), surgeon to St. Bartholomew's Hospital, London, who is also remembered for his descriptions of fracture-dislocation of the ankle joint and the spinal deformity following tuberculosis of the vertebral column.

D. TRUE An increased incidence of skin cancer is associated with industrial exposure to a wide range of carcinogenic hydrocarbons derived from oil, pitch and tar.

E. TRUE Wood workers in the furniture industry have a high incidence of carcinoma of the nasal sinuses.

Malignant tumours occur with increased frequency in association
with:-

A. duodenal ulcer
B. exstrophy of the bladder
C. osteitis deformans (Paget's disease of bone)
D. osteomyelitis sinus
E. ulcerative colitis.

Raised serum alpha-fetoprotein (AFP) levels are common in association with:-

A. carcinomas of the bladder
B. carcinomas of the breast
C. hepatomas
D. malignant lymphomas
E. malignant teratomas.

Answers overleaf

Tum. 8 Answers

A. FALSE Malignant change does not occur in a duodenal ulcer. By contrast, chronic peptic ulcers of the stomach do undergo malignant change though such transformation is much less common than was formerly supposed—the frequency is probably about one per cent.

B. TRUE Patients with this rare and severe congenital abnormality may survive into adult life and in such cases commonly develop bladder tumours which are usually mucoid adenocarcinomas.

C. TRUE Osteitis deformans undoubtedly predisposes to the development of osteosarcoma, though the frequency is difficult to establish. Most osteosarcomas arise in the age group 10 – 25 years but there is a second, smaller, peak of incidence in persons over 50 years of age when it arises as a complication of osteitis deformans.

D. TRUE Squamous cell carcinoma of the skin at the edge of a chronic osteomyelitis sinus is a well recognised but uncommon complication.

E. TRUE Patients with a long history of ulcerative colitis are particularly prone to develop adenocarcinomas of the colon or rectum. Usually the colitis has been present for at least ten years before tumours develop: they are highly malignant tumours, often multiple, and many of them are mucoid adenocarcinomas.

Tum. 9 Answers

A. B. C. D. & E. FALSE, FALSE, TRUE, FALSE, and **TRUE** Alpha-fetoprotein (AFP) is produced by yolk sac and tissues of the fetal liver and gastrointestinal tract. Small amounts of AFP in the plasma can be found in association with many types of malignant tumour but high levels are a common finding only in association with hepatomas and malignant teratomas (especially those with yolk sac components). Significant levels of AFP have not been found with carcinomas of the bladder and breasts or with malignant lymphomas.

Tumours occurring more commonly in children than in adults include:-

A. acute leukaemia
B. malignant melanoma
C. nephroblastoma (Wilms' tumour)
D. neuroblastoma
E. osteoclastoma (giant cell tumour of bone).

Osteosarcomas:-

A. commonly arise in the metaphysis of long bones
B. commonly invade joints
C. are a complication of osteitis deformans (Paget's disease)
D. have a peak incidence in patients between 10 and 25 years old
E. spread chiefly by lymphatics.

Phaeochromocytomas may be associated with:-

A. paroxysmal hypertension
B. persistent hypertension
C. glycosuria
D. a familial incidence
E. medullary carcinoma of the thyroid.

Answers overleaf

Tum. 10 Answers

A. TRUE   Leukaemia has a wide age distribution but there is a relatively high incidence of the acute form in children and of the chronic form in older people.

B. FALSE   This is an uncommon tumour in childhood.

C. & D. TRUE   Both these tumours typically occur in early childhood as also does the cerebellar medulloblastoma. They are all rare in adults.

D. FALSE   This tumour rarely occurs in patients under the age of 20 years.

Tum. 11 Answers

A. TRUE   About threequarters of all cases occur in the long bones of the legs and arms: about half of the cases occur around the knee.

B. FALSE   Joint cavities are rarely invaded.

C. & D. TRUE   About threequarters of all patients are aged 10 to 25: many of the remaining cases are in much older patients with osteitis deformans.

D. FALSE   Distant spread is mainly by the blood stream. Lymphatic spread does occur but is uncommon.

Tum. 12 Answers

A. & B. TRUE   These tumours are usually and typically associated with paroxysmal hypertension, but they can also produce sustained hypertension.

C. TRUE   Glycosuria is common and diabetes mellitus occurs in a significant proportion of cases.

D. TRUE   There is sometimes a familial incidence, especially in those patients with associated neurofibromatosis or other endocrine tumours.

E. TRUE   There is an association between these two tumours especially in familial cases, and other endocrine tumours may also be present. This is another example of the multiple endocrine adenoma syndrome (see also question Syst. 3)—not entirely a happy title as in some instances, such as the present one, not all the tumours are benign.

246

3. OTHER GENERAL PATHOLOGY

Increased melanin pigmentation of the skin occurs in:-

A. adrenocortical failure (Addison's disease)
B. arsenic poisoning
C. haemochromatosis
D. hypopituitarism
E. neurofibromatosis.

Diseases transmitted by autosomal recessive genes include:-

A. cystic fibrosis of the pancreas
B. familial adenomatous polyposis (polyposis coli)
C. haemophilia
D. hereditary spherocytosis
E. red-green colour blindness.

Answers overleaf

Gen. 1 Answers

A. TRUE A general increase in skin pigmentation occurs especially in normally pigmented areas and in those exposed to irritation or sunlight. Pigmentation also occurs on the buccal mucosa and sides of the tongue. Increased secretion of pituitary melanocyte-stimulating hormone occurs when the normal suppressing action of the adrenal wanes with destruction of the adrenal cortex.

B. TRUE In chronic arsenical poisoning a characteristic stippled pigmentation occurs.

C. TRUE This condition is also known as 'bronzed diabetes'. The skin shows haemosiderosis and increased melanin pigmentation.

D. FALSE In this case there is no question of the pituitary being overactive.

E. TRUE *Cafe-au-lait spots* on the skin, large melanin-pigmented macules, are quite common in neurofibromatosis (von Recklinghausen's disease).

Gen. 2 Answers

A. TRUE Cystic fibrosis is one of the commonest single-gene inherited disorders with an incidence in Caucasians of about 1 in 2,000 live births.

B. FALSE This rare disease is transmitted by a dominant gene.

C. FALSE The classical form of haemophilia (haemophilia A) is due to a deficiency of factor VIII (anti-haemophilic globulin). It is an uncommon condition but it is by far the commonest of the inherited defects of coagulation. It is inherited as a sex-linked recessive character and the peccant gene is located on the X chromosome. The disorder is transmitted by females and manifested in males. Haemophilia in the female is excessively rare but can occur with the homozygous state or in the XO form of Turner's syndrome. The much less common *Christmas disease* (haemophilia B—factor IX deficiency) has a similar mode of inheritance.

D. FALSE This relatively common form of haemolytic anaemia is inherited as an autosomal dominant character (see also Question Haem. 1 Answer B).

E. FALSE This common form of colour blindness is inherited as a sex-linked recessive character.

Exposure to ionising radiation can produce:-

A. fibrosis
B. leukaemia
C. squamous cell carcinoma
D. telangiectasia
E. thrombocytopenia.

Amyloid deposition occurs in association with:-

A. medullary carcinoma of the thyroid
B. multiple myeloma
C. repeated blood transfusions
D. rheumatic fever
E. rheumatoid arthritis.

Answers overleaf

Gen. 3 Answers

A. TRUE   Ionising radiation produces a chronic inflammatory reaction with consequent fibrosis. Thus radiotherapy of abdominal lymph nodal metastases of a seminoma has led to renal fibrosis and subsequent development of malignant hypertension, and pulmonary fibrosis is an occasional complication of radiotherapy for breast cancer.

B. TRUE   An increased incidence of leukaemia has been recorded in patients with ankylosing spondylitis treated by radiotherapy and in survivors of the atomic bomb attacks on Hiroshima and Nagasaki.

C. TRUE   There is a well established association between irradiation of the skin and the subsequent development of skin cancer.

D. TRUE   Thin-walled blood vessels commonly develop in irradiated skin.

E. TRUE   Whole body irradiation can cause severe bone marrow damage with depression of red cell, white cell and platelet formation. The thrombocytopenia can produce a severe haemorrhagic state and death may result from massive haemorrhage.

Gen. 4 Answers

A. TRUE   This uncommon tumour arises from the para-follicular (C) cells of the thyroid. It consists of solid sheets of tumour cells set in a hyaline stroma which often contains abundant amyloid. Tumours of other apud cells may also exhibit stromal amyloid deposits.

B. TRUE   Amyloidosis develops in about ten per cent of patients with these plasma cell tumours.

C. & D. FALSE   There is no increased incidence of amyloidosis.

E. TRUE   Formerly chronic suppuration was the main cause of amyloidosis. Nowa... ys die commonest cause is probably rheumatoid arthritis.

250

Hypertrophy of an organ or tissue can be caused by:-

A. amyloid infiltration
B. damage to the nerve supply
C. increased blood supply
D. increased functional demand
E. the action of toxins.

Hyperplasia can occur in:-

A. heart muscle
B. nerve cells
C. smooth muscle
D. the breasts
E. the parathyroids.

Answers overleaf

Gen. 5 Answers

A. FALSE Amyloid infiltration can cause enlargement of an organ but not hypertrophy.

B. FALSE Nerve damage will produce disuse atrophy.

C. FALSE There may be enlargement due to congestion but not hypertrophy.

D. TRUE Hypertrophy of an organ or tissue is due to increase in size of individual cells. In pure hypertrophy there is no proliferation of specialised cells. It is rarely seen except in muscle and the stimulus is almost always mechanical.

E. FALSE Toxins tend to produce tissue damage and never produce hypertrophy.

Gen. 6 Answers

A. B. & C. FALSE Muscle and nerve cells are unable to multiply in postnatal life. Increase in size of muscle is due to hypertrophy.

D. & E. TRUE Hyperplasia is the increase in size of an organ or tissue due to an increase in number of cells. It occurs only in tissues capable of proliferation. The main causal factors are increased work load or endocrine stimulation.

252

Intracellular haemosiderin deposition is found in association with:-

A. haemochromatosis
B. haemolytic anaemia
C. heart failure
D. infarction
E. repeated blood transfusions.

A high protein content is characteristic of the oedema fluid associated with:-

A. acute inflammation
B. allergic oedema
C. cardiac failure
D. famine (nutritional oedema)
E. the nephrotic syndrome.

Answers overleaf

Gen. 7 Answers

A. TRUE In this rare condition a heavy and progressive deposition of haemosiderin occurs in many parts of the body, and in some of the affected organs, e.g. liver and pancreas, extensive destructive fibrosis occurs. Although the disease only becomes clinically apparent in middle age it is due to an inborn error of iron metabolism. In addition to haemosiderin deposition there may be excessive deposition of two iron-free pigments: melanin in the skin and the 'wear and tear' pigment lipofuscin in many tissues.

B. TRUE In all types of haemolytic anaemia there is increased red cell destruction: liberated haemoglobin is broken down by cells of the reticulo-endothelial system into haemosiderin and bilirubin. The haemosiderin is stored mainly in reticulo-endothelial cells in the liver, spleen and bone marrow, but is also found in parenchymal cells of the liver and kidney.

C. TRUE In the congested lungs of the left ventricular failure small haemorrhages occur. Haemosiderin from red cell breakdown is ingested by alveolar macrophages—and the so-called heart-failure cells.

D. TRUE All infarcts contain some blood and in the reparative phase scavenging macrophages ingest cell debris—and this includes haemosiderin.

E. TRUE The process here is essentially similar to that in a haemolytic anaemia (see B above).

Gen. 8 Answers

A. & B. TRUE In both cases there is an increased vascular permeability so that a protein-rich exudate forms with free passage of plasma protein into the extravascular compartment. Inflammatory exudates commonly contain $2-4$ g per 100 ml. of protein and sometimes have as much as plasma ($6-7$ g per 100 ml).

C. D. & E. FALSE In all these conditions the oedema fluid is a true transudate with a protein content of less than 1 g per 100 ml. The causation of oedema in cardiac failure is still not fully elucidated, but there are two important factors: firstly, venous and capillary pressure are raised and secondly, there is a failure of renal sodium excretion, so that both sodium and water are retained in the body. The oedema of famine and of the nephrotic syndrome are due to hypoproteinaemia.

Air embolism is a complication of:-

A. artificial respiration
B. *Clostridium welchii* infections
C. deep sea diving
D. intravenous therapy
E. operations on the head and neck.

Thrombus formation is favoured by:-

A. damage to vascular endothelium
B. slowing of blood flow
C. increased platelet count
D. heparin therapy
E. oestrogen therapy.

Answers overleaf

Gen. 9 Answers

A. FALSE   Unless a most exceptional degree of force was used which might cause major chest injury.

B. FALSE   Gas bubbles may form in the blood after death as the result of *Clostridium welchii* proliferation, but this is not air embolism.

C. TRUE   A special form of air embolism (decompression sickness or Caisson disease) occurs in workers exposed to high atmospheric pressures. It is thus seen in underwater construction workers and divers. The increased atmospheric pressure causes increased solution of air in the blood stream. If return to normal pressure is too rapid air escapes from solution as gas bubbles: although oxygen and carbon dioxide are rapidly reabsorbed, bubbles of the less soluble nitrogen persist.

D. TRUE   It can occur when positive pressure is used in blood transfusions; by injecting drugs into the tubing of an intravenous infusion; during haemodialysis; and when using central venous catheters.

E. TRUE   The inadvertent opening of a large vein may allow air to be sucked in.

Gen. 10 Answers

A. B. & C. TRUE   These constitute Virchow's triad—the three factors basic to thrombosis. The last component of the triad—increased coagulability of the blood—is predominantly due to platelet factors, namely an increase in their number and in their adhesiveness. Virchow (1821—1902) was the most famous pathologist of all time and his Institute of Pathology in Berlin, where he spent 46 years, was a world centre for research: he taught that the cell is the seat of disease and his *Cellular Pathologie* published in 1858 is one of the really great books in the history of medicine.

D. FALSE   Heparin is an anticoagulant.

E. TRUE   The oral contraceptive pill is associated with an increased incidence of thrombosis. Oestrogen is the responsible component and progesterone does not appear to have any effect.

4. MICROBIOLOGY

Lesions resulting from *Streptococcus pyogenes* **infection include:-**

A. acute proliferative glomerulonephritis
B. acute osteomyelitis
C. acute tonsillitis
D. lobar pneumonia
E. rheumatic fever.

Answers overleaf

Micro. 1 Answers

A. TRUE   Typically there is a *Streptococcus pyogenes* infection of the throat, upper respiratory tract or middle ear, one to three weeks before the onset of renal disease. Not all strains of *Streptococcus pyogenes* are nephritogenic; the most important are Griffiths types 12 and 49. This type of nephritis is essentially an immune-complex disease; circulating antigen—antibody complexes become trapped in the glomerular basement membrane and excite an inflammatory reaction.

B. FALSE   *Staphylococcus pyogenes* is the most important causal agent in acute osteomyelitis.

C. TRUE   *Streptococcus pyogenes* is present in the throats of about 10 per cent of people and is a common cause of tonsillitis.

D. FALSE   This disease is due to infection with the pneumococcus—*Streptococcus pneumoniae*.

E. TRUE   Rheumatic fever can follow infection by any strain of *Streptococcus pyogenes*. There is an interval of one to three weeks between the initial infection (usually tonsillitis) and the appearance of cardiac and joint lesions. The exact pathogenesis is still unknown but there is probably an allergic basis: it has been shown that cross-reacting antigens exist between streptococcal products and both cardiac muscle and heart valves.

Streptococcus viridans **infection is a major cause of:-**

A. food poisoning
B. scarlet fever
C. skin infections
D. subacute bacterial endocarditis
E. urinary tract infections.

Staphylococcus aureus **can produce:-**

A. coagulase
B. enterotoxin
C. haemolysin
D. leucocidin
E. penicillinase.

Answers overleaf

Micro. 2 Answers

A. FALSE   Most outbreaks of food poisoning are due to infection with salmonella species or to ingestion of preformed toxin produced by strains of *Staphylococcus aureus* or *Clostridium welchii*.

B. FALSE   This disease, now uncommon, is the result of infection with strains of *Streptococcus pyogenes* producing erythrogenic toxin.

C. FALSE   *Staphylococcus aureus* is the most important organism in this respect.

D. TRUE   *Streptococcus viridans* is an organism of relatively low virulence. It is commonly an inhabitant of the normal mouth or throat. In patients with periodontal disease or following tooth extraction bacteraemia may occur: usually these organisms are dealt with by the normal body defences, but in patients with damaged heart valves (rheumatic or congenital heart disease) organisms may settle and multiply.

E. FALSE   A wide range of organisms produce these infections and, of these, *Escherichia coli* is the most common. *Streptococcus viridans* is a very rare cause.

Micro. 3 Answers

A. TRUE   Coagulase is a diffusible protein which converts soluble fibrinogen into insoluble fibrin. It is produced by pathogenic staphylococci and its presence is used as the specific defining feature of *Staphylococcus aureus* irrespective of pigment production by the organism.

B. TRUE   Some strains produce enterotoxin: they are an important cause of food poisoning.

C. TRUE   A wide range of haemolysins are produced by various strains.

D. TRUE   Most strains produce a powerful toxin that is able to destroy white blood cells.

E. TRUE   Nearly all strains of *Staphylococcus aureus* found in hospital that are penicillin-resistant produce penicillinase.

Organisms that grow only under strictly anaerobic conditions include:-

A. *Actinomyces israeli*
B. *Clostridium tetani*
C. *Clostridium welchii*
D. *Escherichia coli*
E. *Pseudomonas aeruginosa.*

Organisms that can be cultivated under aerobic conditions in media *not* containing living cells include:-

A. herpes viruses
B. influenza virus
C. *Mycobacterium tuberculosis*
D. *Neisseria gonorrhoeae*
E. *Treponema pallidum.*

Answers overleaf

Micro. 4 Answers

A. B. & C. TRUE All these organisms are strict anaerobes together with all other species of *Clostridium* and anaerobic streptococci.

D. & E. FALSE These organisms will grow under aerobic or anaerobic conditions.

Micro. 5 Answers

A. & B. FALSE Viruses are obligatory intracellular parasites—they can grow and reproduce only in living cells. In addition to laboratory animals, the developing chick embryo and tissue culture are used for the growth and isolation of viruses.

C. TRUE This organism is grown with difficulty in artificial media and even in special enriched media growth is slow. Usually it is cultured on a coagulated egg medium, e.g. Dorset's egg medium or a modified form of it such as Löwenstein-Jensen medium which has certain additives to encourage growth, and even then 3 – 6 weeks may be needed for colonies to appear.

D. TRUE This organism is also difficult to grow and an enriched medium such as 'chocolate' (heated blood) agar is required. Growth can be enhanced by incubation in an atmosphere containing 5 – 10 per cent carbon dioxide.

E. FALSE This organism cannot be cultured on artificial media.

Organisms producing exotoxin include:-

A. *Clostridium welchii*
B. *Corynebacterium diphtheriae*
C. *Escherichia coli*
D. *Pseudomonas aeruginosa*
E. *Streptococcus pyogenes.*

Blood culture is a useful diagnostic procedure in:-

A. infective endocarditis
B. miliary tuberculosis
C. rheumatic fever
D. secondary syphilis
E. typhoid fever.

Answers overleaf

Micro. 6 Answers

A. TRUE   All the pathogenic clostridia produce powerful exotoxins. Cl. welchii produces at least eight toxins: the most important is the alpha-toxin which has great haemolytic and necrotizing activity.

B. TRUE   Although a diphtheritic membrane in the larynx or trachea may produce respiratory obstruction, the main complications of diphtheria are due to the action of circulating exotoxin. Hence antitoxin is of value in treatment and toxoids provide effective active immunity.

C. & D. FALSE   These organisms produce endotoxins but not exotoxins. They are both important organisms in relation to Gram negative bacteraemia (endotoxic or bacteraemic shock) in which sudden collapse may occur in a patient following the entry into the blood steam of large numbers of Gram-negative bacilli. This condition is often brought about by some manipulation or operative procedure on the bladder or urethra.

E. TRUE   Some strains produce an erythrogenic toxin responsible for the rash of scarlet fever.

Micro. 7 Answers

A. TRUE   A most important procedure. The sample should be divided into three parts and incubated (in an appropriate medium) aerobically, aerobically plus 5 – 10 per cent carbon dioxide and anaerobically. It may be necessary to repeat the blood culture several times before a positive result is obtained.

B. FALSE   Although this is a blood borne infection the organism cannot be recovered from the blood.

C. FALSE   Organisms are not present in the blood or heart lesions. The disease follows 2 – 4 weeks after a *Streptococcus pyogenes* infection—usually tonsillitis; it is an example of an immune-complex reaction, a hypersensitivity response by the affected tissues to circulating streptococcal products.

D. FALSE   The organism cannot be cultured.

E. TRUE   In all forms of enteric fever blood culture is extremely valuable and is most likely to be positive early in the illness.

Metastatic pyaemic abscesses are a feature of infection with:-

A. *Brucella abortus*
B. *Clostridium tetani*
C. *Corynebacterium diphtheriae*
D. *Staphylococcus aureus*
E. *Streptococcus viridans.*

The effects of virus diseases in humans include the production of:-

A. antibodies
B. congenital defects
C. inclusion bodies
D. interferon
E. multinucleate giant cells.

Answers overleaf

Micro. 8 Answers

A. FALSE   This organism enters the circulation but the tissue reaction at the site of lodgement is a granuloma and not an abscess.

B. & C. FALSE   The ill effects of these organisms are not due to bacteraemia but to a powerful exotoxin.

D. TRUE   Metastatic abscesses are an important complication of infections with *Staph. aureus.*

E. FALSE   *Strep. viridans* infections can cause bacteraemia leading to subacute bacterial endocarditis with embolic phenomena, but it does not yield pyaemic abscesses.

Micro. 9 Answers

A. TRUE   All viruses are antigenic and induce the formation of specific antibodies. These antibodies are important in combating viral infections and in the development of immunity.

B. TRUE   The classical example is rubella (German measles). Women contracting rubella in the first trimester of pregnancy have a high incidence of deformed children—about 25 per cent. A wide range of deformities may result including heart lesions, microcephaly, cataracts and deafness.

C. TRUE   Some viruses produce intracellular masses visible on light microscopy. These inclusion bodies may consist of aggregated virus particles or they may represent products of degeneration of the host cell. They may be intranuclear, e.g. the large bodies seen in cytomegalovirus infection, or they may be in the cytoplasm, e.g. the Negri bodies in the neurons of patients with rabies.

D. TRUE   Interferons are a group of proteins produced by cells infected with virus. They make the cells resistant to further infection. Unfortunately their promise as therapeutic agents has not been maintained.

E. TRUE   The outstanding example is the Warthin-Finkeldy giant cell of measles (see Infl. 1).

The glandular fever (infectious mononucleosis) syndrome can be produced by:-

A. adenoviruses
B. cytomegalovirus
C. Epstein-Barr virus
D. rhinoviruses
E. *Toxoplasma gondii.*

Answers overleaf

Micro. 10 Answers

A. FALSE These viruses are associated with a wide range of respiratory tract illnesses, conjunctivitis and adenitis, but they do not produce mononucleosis in the blood with atypical lymphocytes.

B. TRUE Cytomegalovirus infection can produce a persistent fever with a marked mononucleosis with atypical lymphocytes. The Paul-Bunnell reaction is, however, negative. This infection can be transmitted by blood transfusions, usually with an incubation of 4 – 6 weeks.

C. TRUE This is the usual causal agent and these cases usually produce a positive Paul-Bunnell reaction.

D. FALSE These are the common cold viruses.

E. TRUE Latent infection with this organism is common. When overt disease occurs in children or adults it produces a glandular fever-like illness with lymphocytosis. The Paul-Bunnell reaction is negative. Occasionally severe forms of the disease occur: congenital toxoplasmosis, acquired *in utero* from an infected mother, can cause major cerebral damage with encephalitis and hydrocephalus.

5. IMMUNOLOGY

Living vaccines are used in immunization against:-

A. diphtheria
B. poliomyelitis
C. tetanus
D. tuberculosis
E. typhoid fever.

Thymus-dependent lymphocytes (T lymphocytes) are:-

A. actively phagocytic
B. associated with cell-mediated immunity
C. precursors of plasma cells
D. the predominant type of blood lymphocyte
E. shorter lived than bursa-dependent lymphocytes (B lymphocytes).

Answers overleaf

Imm. 1 Answers

A. FALSE   Active immunization with diphtheria toxoid is used.

B. TRUE   Sabin oral vaccine consists of attenuated living viruses of types 1, 2 and 3. Also effective is the Salk vaccine which contains the same three types of killed polioviruses.

C. FALSE   Tetanus toxoid is used in immunization.

D. TRUE   BCG (Bacille Calmette-Guérin) is an attenuated bovine strain of *Mycobacterium tuberculosis*.

E. FALSE   TAB vaccine is a suspension of killed organisms (*Salmonella typhi* and *Salmonella paratyphi* A and B).

Imm. 2 Answers

A. B. & C. FALSE TRUE and FALSE   Lymphocytes have no significant phagocytic activity. In birds there are two main primary lymphoid organs, the thymus and the cloacal bursa (bursa of Fabricius), in which lymphocyte precursors are prepared for their later immunological functions. Two series of cells arise: T lymphocytes (thymus-dependent lymphocytes) and B lymphocytes (bursa-dependent or thymus-independent lymphocytes) with quite distinct functions. In man, and all mammals, there is no cloacal bursa and the site is still debated—whether it be lymphoid tissue of the gastrointestinal mucosa or of the bone marrow; nevertheless the terms T and B lymphocytes are retained in human pathology. T cells are responsible for cell-mediated immunity. B cells are responsible for immunoglobulin synthesis and the production of humoral antibodies; plasma cells are derived from B lymphocytes.

D. TRUE   The great majority of lymphocytes found in the blood are T cells; about 15% of small lymphocytes in the peripheral blood are B cells.

E. FALSE   T cells have a much longer life than B cells and can survive for months or years.

Plasma cells:-

A. are actively phagocytic
B. are concerned with antibody production
C. are derived from bursa-dependent lymphocytes (B lymphocytes).
D. contain abundant histamine
E. contain abundant rough endoplasmic reticulum.

Plasma gamma globulin (immunoglobulin) is raised in:-

A. cirrhosis of the liver
B. diabetes mellitus
C. sarcoidosis
D. systemic lupus erythematosus
E. the nephrotic syndrome.

Answers overleaf

Imm. 3 Answers

A. FALSE   Plasma cells, like their precursor lymphocytes, have no significant phagocytic activity.

B, & C. TRUE   When B lymphocytes are exposed to antigen many of them differentiate into plasma cells which synthesise the appropriate antibody.

D. FALSE   Mast cells and basophils are the major souces of histamine in man. Very small amounts may be present in the plasma cells.

E. TRUE   The abundant endoplasmic reticulum in plasma cells indicates that they are actively engaged in protein synthesis (mainly immunoglobulin).

Imm. 4 Answers

A. TRUE   The liver is the site of synthesis of most of the plasma proteins—but not gamma globulins. In cirrhosis of the liver there is a fall in plasma albumin; in contrast the gamma globulin level in the plasma is raised though the cause is not yet clear.

B. FALSE   In severe diabetes with renal complications and the nephrotic syndrome, the plasma gamma globulin is reduced.

C. TRUE   The cause is not known.

D. TRUE   Hypergammaglobulinaemia is a feature of auto-immune disorders such as systemic lupus erythematosus and rheumatoid arthritis.

E. FALSE   The plasma gamma globulin is reduced partly due to urinary loss.

Complications of renal transplantation include:-

A. an increased incidence of infection
B. an increased incidence of malignant tumours
C. dense infiltration of the renal cortex by lymphoid cells
D. fibrinoid necrosis of renal arterioles
E. intimal proliferation of renal arteries.

Answers overleaf

Imm. 5 Answers

A. TRUE The main problem in organ transplantation is the prevention of graft rejection. To reduce the risk of rejection immunosuppressive drugs are given, but their usage is associated with an increased susceptibility to infection both with virulent pathogens and with opportunistic organisms such as candida and other fungal species, cytomegalovirus and *Pneumocystis carinii*.

B. TRUE There is an increased incidence of a wide range of cancers, and in particular of malignant lymphomas, in patients who have had renal or cardiac transplants. It is probably a consequence of the use of immunosuppressive drugs.

C. D. & E. TRUE All these changes can occur in the transplanted kidney and are indicators of rejection. In one form of acute rejection there is a dense infiltration of the cortex by lymphoid cells. This cell-mediated reaction is usually diminished by immunosuppressive treatment. Patients receiving immunosuppressive drugs more often show a humoral form of acute rejection with necrotic lesions of arterioles and small arteries. Chronic rejection, months or years after transplantation, is associated with severe arterial narrowing due to intimal proliferation.

Diagnostic tests based on an agglutination reaction include:-

A. Coomb's test
B. Mantoux test
C. Paul-Bunnell test
D. Wasserman reaction
E. Widal reaction.

Answers overleaf

A. TRUE In this test red blood cells coated with IgG can be agglutinated by antibody against IgG (antiglobulin or Coombs's reagent). The *direct* test demonstrates globulin already absorbed onto red cells and is of value in detecting haemolytic anaemias due to antibodies. The *indirect* test is used in cross-matching blood; it is a more complicated test and detects the presence in a patient's serum of incomplete antibody—that is antibody which is unable to agglutinate red cells directly.

B. FALSE This test is an example of a hypersensitivity reaction—the tuberculin reaction. It is a test for cell-mediated immunity in which a small quantity of tuberculoprotein is injected intradermally. In a sensitised person a raised erythematous patch develops in 24 hours and persists for several days.

C. TRUE In the classical type of infectious mononucleosis (glandular fever) many patients develop heterophil agglutinins for sheep red cells in their blood. These agglutinins are demonstrated by the Paul-Bunnell test. In the type of infectious mononucleosis due to cytomegalovirus infection the Paul-Bunnell test is negative.

D. FALSE This test is based on complement fixation.

E. TRUE The Frenchman Widal (1862 – 1929) introduced this test in 1896 to diagnose typhoid fever. It is the first example of a diagnostic serological test. The serum of patients with enteric fever will cause agglutination in a suspension of typhoid bacilli.

6. HAEMATOLOGY

Haemolysis is a feature of:-

A. haemophilia
B. hereditary spherocytosis
C. sickle cell disease
D. thalassaemia
E. thrombocytopenic purpura.

An iron deficiency anaemia due to chronic blood loss is characterised by a raised:-

A. mean cell haemoglobin (MCH)
B. mean cell volume (MCV)
C. plasma bilirubin concentration
D. plasma iron concentration
E. white blood cell count.

Answers overleaf

Haem. 1 Answers

A. FALSE   This is a haemorrhagic disorder due to a coagulation defect. It is characterised by a congenital deficiency in production of antihaemophilic globulin (Factor VIII). Haemolysis is not a feature.

B. TRUE   Spherocytes have an abnormal cell membrane: they accumulate in the spleen where they are phagocytosed and destroyed. Splenectomy often abolishes the haemolytic process, but does not affect the red cell malformation.

C. & D. TRUE   These disorders of haemoglobin synthesis are genetically determined. In the homozygous state (sickle cell disease and thalassaemia major) haemolysis is often severe: the affected red cells are mechanically fragile and are destroyed in the circulation.

E. FALSE   This is a haemorrhagic disorder due to a low platelet count. Haemolysis is not a feature. The thrombocytopenia may be primary or secondary. The causes of secondary thrombocytopenia are many and include other blood disorders, e.g. leukaemia; exposure to drugs, e.g. 'sedormid'; and exposure to physical agents, e.g. ionising radiation.

Haem. 2 Answers

A. FALSE   The cells are not saturated with haemoglobin so that the mean cell haemoglobin is reduced below 27 pg (the normal range for MCH is 29 ± 2 pg). The anaemia is typically hypochromic and in blood films from severe cases the poorly haemoglobinised red cells appear as rings.

B. FALSE   The anaemia is typically microcytic: the red cells have a smaller diameter than normal and a reduced volume (the normal range for MCV is 87 ± 5 fl).

C. FALSE   There is no evidence of haemolysis.

D. FALSE   In severe or longstanding cases the serum iron is low.

E. FALSE   The white cell count is usually normal, though immediately following a major haemorrhage there may be a transient leucocytosis.

Haemolytic anaemias are characterised by:-

A. an increased incidence of gall stones
B. a reduced life span of red blood cells
C. jaundice
D. leucopenia
E. reticulocytosis.

Answers overleaf

Haem. 3 Answers

A. TRUE   The increased red blood cell destruction leads to an increased excretion of bilirubin via the bile which in turn predisposes to the formation of pigment stones in the gall bladder.

B. TRUE   The increase in rate of red blood cell destruction is automatically linked with a decrease in life span of the cells. The life span of red blood cells can now be accurately measured by labelling the cells with radioactive isotopes (e.g. ^{51}Cr, ^{59}Fe or ^{14}C) and following their fate in serial blood samples (the normal life span is about 120 days).

C. TRUE   Haemolytic anaemia and haemolytic jaundice (acholuric jaundice) are essentially synonymous. The haemolysis leads to the production of bilirubin in excess of the amount that the liver can excrete so that the serum level rises and clinical jaundice results.

D. FALSE   The white blood cell count is usually unaffected, though in an acute haemolytic episode there may be a transient leucocytosis.

E. TRUE   In haemolytic diseases red cell production by the bone marrow is increased and there is an outpouring of young red cells into the circulation, the reticulocyte count is always increased and may reach high levels (10 − 20 per cent compared with a normal of under one per cent): after a haemolytic crisis even higher levels occur (30 per cent or more).

Pernicious (Addisonian) anaemia is associated with:-

A. vitamin B_{12} deficiency
B. folic acid deficiency
C. leucopenia
D. atrophic gastritis
E. an increased incidence of gastric carcinoma.

Answers overleaf

281

Haem. 4 Answers

A. TRUE   This disease is the most important type of vitamin B_{12} deficiency. The basic lesion is an atrophic gastritis probably of autoimmune origin: as a result intrinsic factor, which is produced by gastric parietal cells and is essential for vitamin B_{12} absorption, is no longer produced. The clinical features were first described in 1855 by Addison (1793 – 1860, physician at Guy's hospital, London, who also gave the first clinical description of chronic adrenocortical failure—see Gen. 3 A. It is noteworthy that both these conditions have an organ-specific autoimmune origin).

B. FALSE   Folic acid deficiency produces a megaloblastic anaemia but is not associated with the gastric and neurological features of pernicious anaemia.

C. TRUE   Neutropenia and also thrombocytopenia occur.

D. TRUE   Severe atrophic gastritis or gastric atrophy is the basic lesion. It affects all layers of the stomach wall in the fundus and body portions and leads to a histamine-fast achlorhydria as well as the failure to produce intrinsic factor.

E. TRUE   There is an above average incidence of gastric carcinoma in patients with pernicious anaemia.

Secondary polycythaemia can be a feature of:-

A. chronic lung disease
B. congenital heart disease
C. primary gastric carcinoma
D. primary renal carcinoma
E. the 'blind-loop' syndrome.

Neutrophil leucocytosis is a feature of:-

A. crush injuries
B. hypersplenism
C. lobar pneumonia
D. myocardial infarction
E. whooping cough (pertussis).

Answers overleaf

Haem. 5 Answers

A. & B. TRUE The most important cause of secondary polycythaemia is hypoxia resulting from chronic lung disease, congenital heart disease with right-to-left shunts, and residence at high altitude.

C. FALSE Patients with gastric carcinoma are usually anaemic.

D. TRUE Renal production of erythropoietin may occur in many forms of chronic renal disease including carcinoma and give rise to polycythaemia. More usually in renal cell carcinoma bleeding occurs to produce an iron-deficiency anaemia.

E. FALSE Any form of prolonged intestinal stasis may lead to abnormal bacterial proliferation and an abnormal uptake of vitamin B_{12} by them—so producing megaloblastic anaemia.

Haem. 6 Answers

A. TRUE A moderate neutrophil leucocytosis occurs with any severe degree of tissue injury, even in the absence of infection.

B. FALSE In many forms of splenomegaly there is a reduction in number of circulating white blood cells and sometimes also of red cells and platelets. The exact mechanism is not known, but in part at least it is due to pooling in, and increased destruction of blood cells within, the enlarged spleen.

C. TRUE A neutrophil leucocytosis is the typical reaction to pyogenic infection and most other bacterial infections.

D. TRUE Any substantial degree of tissue necrosis, whatever the cause, is associated with a moderate neutrophil leucocytosis.

E. FALSE The typical reaction here is a lymphocytic leucocytosis.

Leucopenia is often associated with:-

A. acute leukaemia
B. exposure to ionising radiation
C. overwhelming bacterial infection
D. parasitic infestation
E. typhoid fever.

Human blood platelets:-

A. contain 5-hydroxytryptamine
B. contain heparin
C. do not have a nucleus
D. help to initiate thrombus formation
E. are necessary for clot retraction.

Answers overleaf

Haem. 7 Answers

A. TRUE   A considerable number of patients at some stage of the disease exhibit a neutropenia—the so-called aleukaemic stage. Severe anaemia and thrombocytopenia also occur.

B. TRUE   Bone marrow damage follows total body irradiation with reduction in all types of blood cell.

C. TRUE   The usual response to bacterial infection is leucocytosis but in a very severe infection neutropenia can occur and is a serious prognostic sign.

D. FALSE   The usual response to parasitic infestations is an eosinophilia.

E. TRUE   A mild leucopenia is seen in typhoid fever: it does not usually occur in paratyphoid infections.

Haem. 8 Answers

A. TRUE   Most of the blood 5-hydroxytryptamine is adsorbed on the platelets.

B. FALSE   Heparin is present in the granules of mast cells.

C. TRUE   Platelets $(2-4\,\mu m$ diameter) do not have a nucleus: they are formed by detachment of cytoplasmic fragments from megakaryocytes—very large cells (up to $100\,\mu m$ diameter) with an irregular lobed nucleus.

D. TRUE   Deposition of platelets on the intimal surface of a damaged blood vessel is the first step in thrombus formation.

E. TRUE   In the absence of platelets clot formation is impaired: any clot formed is soft and retraction is defective.

Purpura is an important manifestation of:-

A. acute leukaemia
B. haemophilia
C. severe infections
D. thrombocytopenia
E. vitamin C deficiency.

A prolonged bleeding time is a feature of:-

A. vitamin C deficiency
B. thrombocytopenic purpura
C. disseminated intravascular coagulation
D. haemophilia
E. Christmas disease.

Answers overleaf

Haem. 9 Answers

A. TRUE   Purpura is a common and important feature of acute leukaemia due to the associated severe thrombocytopenia.

B. FALSE   Purpura is uncommon and not a major feature of disorders of clotting.

C. TRUE   Many severe infections are accompanied by purpura. The platelet count may be normal in such cases and the petechial haemorrhages probably result from toxic damage to capillary walls.

D. TRUE   Purpura is a major feature of all forms of thrombocytopenia.

E. TRUE   The petechial haemorrhages of scurvy are due to vascular damage; the platelet count is usually normal.

Haem. 10 Answers

A. & B. TRUE   The bleeding time is the time taken for a single small skin stab with a sharp needle to stop bleeding. The arrest of bleeding with this minute injury depends on the formation of a platelet thrombus and on capillary wall retraction. Hence bleeding time is prolonged in all purpuric conditions (whether due to thrombocytopenia or to capillary wall damage); it is *not* prolonged in defects of coagulation.

C. TRUE   There are severe defects of coagulation in this condition but because of the consumption of platelets there may also be severe thrombocytopenia.

D. & E. FALSE   In haemophilia A (factor VIII deficiency) and in haemophilia B (Christmas disease—factor IX deficiency) the clotting time is greatly prolonged but the bleeding time is normal.

Complications of blood transfusion include:-

A. cytomegalovirus infection
B. infectious mononucleosis
C. citrate intoxication
D. disseminated intravascular coagulation
E. pulmonary oedema.

Multiple myeloma is often associated with:-

A. a high erythrocyte sedimentation rate
B. hypercalcaemia
C. intercurrent infection
D. renal failure
E. rouleaux formation in blood films.

Answers overleaf

Haem. 11 Answers

A. & B. TRUE Viral hepatitis is a well known complication of blood transfusions; most cases are caused by infectious hepatitis (type A) or serum hepatitis (type B). Other viral infections can also be transmitted and the so-called post-transfusion syndrome—which resembles glandular fever—is usually due to cytomegalovirus or Epstein-Barr virus infection.

C. TRUE Blood for transfusion is stored after addition of an anticoagulant solution which has sodium citrate as a major component. Massive blood transfusion can lead to citrate intoxication and hypocalcaemia.

D. TRUE This is another complication of massive blood transfusion. In stored blood the platelet content and the concentration of several clotting factors rapidly fall. Major transfusions of stored blood may so reduce the patient's levels of platelets and clotting factors as to precipitate disseminated intravascular coagulation.

E. TRUE Too rapid or too big a transfusion can produce pulmonary oedema and congestive heart failure.

Haem. 12 Answers

A. TRUE A greatly raised erythrocyte sedimentation rate, due to hyperglobulinaemia, is characteristic.

B. TRUE A result of the multiple osteolytic bone lesions.

C. TRUE All patients with myeloma have an increased susceptibility to infection but it is especially important in the common IgG myeloma. As a result of abnormal globulin formation the production of other immunoglobulins is impaired.

D. TRUE This is a common and important complication often called myeloma kidney. Several factors contribute to the renal failure, though they may not all operate in an individual case: hypercalcaemia; Bence-Jones protein is precipitated in the renal tubules, blocking them and producing tubular atrophy; direct infiltration of renal substance by myeloma tissue; and the occurrence of amyloidosis.

E. TRUE This again is due to the hyperglobulinaemia.

7. CHEMICAL PATHOLOGY

High gastric acidity is a feature of:-

A. atrophic gastritis
B. carcinoma of stomach
C. duodenal ulcer
D. pernicious anaemia
E. Zollinger-Ellison syndrome.

Hypercalcaemia is a feature of:-

A. acute pancreatitis
B. osteolytic tumour metastases in bone
C. primary hyperparathyroidism
D. sarcoidosis
E. vitamin D intoxication.

A raised plasma alkaline phosphatase level is found in association with:-

A. healing of a fracture
B. hyperparathyroidism
C. obstructive jaundice
D. osteitis deformans (Paget's disease of bone)
E. osteolytic tumour metastases in bone.

Answers overleaf

Chem. 1 Answers

A. & B. FALSE In these conditions the ability of the stomach to secrete acid is normal or subnormal.

C. TRUE On average, patients with duodenal ulcer have a larger parietal cell mass than normal subjects.

D. FALSE In pernicious anaemia there is a complete achlorhydria—the stomach cannot secrete acid even in response to histamine.

E. TRUE A very large and sustained output of acid gastric juice is characteristic of this syndrome. The underlying lesion is a gastrin-secreting tumour (gastrinoma) of pancreatic islet tissue.

Chem. 2 Answers

A. FALSE *Hypo*calcaemia often occurs, probably due to the precipitation of calcium with fatty acids released by enzymatic fat hydrolysis.

B. TRUE A fairly common cause of hypercalcaemia. Calcium is released by local bone destruction from multiple secondary osteolytic deposits.

C. TRUE Excess parathyroid hormone secretion leads to increased mobilisation of calcium from bone.

D. TRUE A rare but well recognised cause of a raised serum calcium. Nephrocalcinosis may occur and lead to death from renal failure.

E. TRUE There is increased intestinal absorption of calcium.

Chem. 3 Answers

A. B. C. & D. TRUE Many cells of the body secrete an alkaline phosphatase and important sites of production include hepatocytes and osteoblasts: excretion occurs in bile and in urine. A raised plasma alkaline phosphatase level can occur as a result of increased secretion or of reduced excretion of the enzyme: thus it can occur in any form of bone disease associated with increased osteoblastic activity or in association with obstruction to the outflow of bile.

E. FALSE Normal plasma levels are found in osteolytic forms of bone disease.

A raised plasma acid phosphatase level is found in association with:-

A. carcinoma of the prostate
B. carcinoma of the rectum
C. hyperparathyroidism
D. obstructive jaundice
E. osteitis deformans (Paget's disease of bone).

A low plasma potassium level is associated with:-

A. aldosterone-secreting tumours of the adrenal (Conn's syndrome)
B. diuretic therapy
C. medullary carcinoma of the thyroid
D. phaeochromocytoma
E. pyloric stenosis.

A raised plasma uric acid level is a feature of:-

A. gout
B. leukaemia
C. myocardial infarction
D. renal failure
E. treatment with cytotoxic drugs.

Answers overleaf

Chem. 4 Answers

A. TRUE Normal and carcinomatous prostatic epithelium secrete an acid phosphatase. Normally this enzyme is secreted into the prostatic fluid, but with invasive carcinoma it enters the blood stream and a high plasma level is found, especially when bony metastases have occurred. The secondary deposits in bone usually cause an osteoblastic reaction so that the plasma alkaline phosphatase is also raised.

B. C. D. & E. FALSE

Chem. 5 Answers

A. TRUE Renal tubular function is altered leading to potassium loss and sodium retention. A similar effect occurs in the secondary aldosteronism associated with nephrosis, cirrhosis or congestive heart failure.

B. TRUE Many diuretics inhibit renal tubular sodium reabsorption and lead to increased urinary potassium loss.

C. FALSE These tumours secrete calcitonin: there is no effect on blood potassium.

D. FALSE These tumours secrete adrenaline and noradrenaline: there is no effect on blood potassium.

E. TRUE Hypokalaemia is most commonly seen in patients with diseases of the gastrointestinal tract associated with diarrhoea and vomiting, resulting in long continued loss of gastrointestinal secretions.

Chem. 6 Answers

A. TRUE In gout there is an increased rate of purine synthesis leading to hyperuricaemia.

B. & C. TRUE Increased tissue breakdown resulting from any cause leads to increased purine catabolism and high plasma urate levels.

D. TRUE In renal failure or urinary tract obstruction, uric acid is retained along with all other urinary constituents.

E. TRUE Increased tissue breakdown occurs.

Hypoglycaemia is a feature of:-

A. adrenocortical failure (Addison's disease)
B. glycogen storage disease
C. haemochromatosis
D. hyperthyroidism
E. patients after gastrectomy.

A raised plasma cholesterol level is a feature of:-

A. chronic biliary obstruction
B. diabetes mellitus
C. haemolytic anaemias
D. myxoedema
E. nephrotic syndrome.

Answers overleaf

Chem. 7 Answers

A. TRUE Hypoglycaemia is an important feature of adreno-cortical failure, but it is often overshadowed by the even more important electrolyte changes—loss of sodium and water and consequent extracellular depletion.

B. TRUE There are several forms of glycogen storage disease, depending on which of a series of enzymes responsible for degrading glycogen is deficient. Hypoglycaemic episodes are a feature of the best known type—von Gierke's disease—and also of many of the other varieties.

C. FALSE Diabetes mellitus often occurs in these patients.

D. FALSE A normal or raised blood sugar is found.

E. TRUE In these patients, after a carbohydrate meal there is abnormally rapid glucose absorption which leads to a high blood sugar level: this in turn stimulates an excessive response of insulin secretion to produce a reactive hypoglycaemia one or two hours after the meal.

Chem. 8 Answers

A. TRUE Failure of cholesterol excretion in the bile leads to a retention hypercholesterolaemia. This occurs in obstructive jaundice and also in forms of hepatitis with an element of intra-hepatic obstruction.

B. TRUE Raised blood levels of fat and cholesterol are common and important.

C. FALSE Hypercholesterolaemia does not occur in pre-hepatic jaundice (see A above).

D. TRUE There is a high plasma cholesterol level which returns to normal when treatment is effective.

E. TRUE Lipaemia and hypercholesterolaemia occur. The reason is unclear.

Prolonged administration of corticosteroids can produce:-

A. glycosuria
B. hypotension
C. muscle wasting
D. osteoporosis
E. suppression of the inflammatory reaction.

Answers overleaf

A. TRUE   The action on carbohydrate metabolism is to produce an insulin-resistant diabetes with hyperglycaemia and glycosuria.

B. FALSE   Hypertension occurs.

C. & D. TRUE   Both these effects result from the catabolic action of corticosteroids on protein metabolism.

E. TRUE   The inflammatory reaction is modified in several ways. There is reduced migration of neutrophils and monocytes. Collagen formation is impaired by reduced fibroblast proliferation and reduced ground substance formation. The immune response is also diminished and antibody production inhibited.

8. SYSTEMIC PATHOLOGY

Precancerous lesions of the large intestine include:-

A. chronic ulcerative colitis
B. diverticular disease
C. familial adenomatous polyposis (polyposis coli)
D. ischaemic colitis
E. villous adenoma.

Peptic ulcers occur in the:-

A. oesophagus
B. jejunum
C. ileum
D. colon
E. rectum.

Answers overleaf

Syst. 1 Answers

A. TRUE Carcinoma of the colon or rectum is an established complication of long-standing ulcerative colitis. Colitis has usually been present for at least ten years before tumours appear. The tumours are highly malignant and often multiple.

B. FALSE

C. TRUE In this rare genetic disorder malignant change almost invariably occurs in one or more of the polyps. The cancers usually develop in early life and are highly malignant.

D. FALSE

E. TRUE Villous adenomas are relatively uncommon but a significant proportion of them undergo malignant change.

Syst. 2 Answers

A. B. C. TRUE Peptic ulcers can occur in any part of the alimentary tract that is directly exposed to the action of hydrochloric acid and pepsin. In the oesophagus peptic ulcers only occur when the lowermost part is lined by gastric mucosa. This can occur with congenital heterotopia or following upgrowth of gastric mucosa in reflux oesophagitis. In the jejunum an *anastomotic ulcer* can develop at the stoma of a gastroenterostomy. When ectopic gastric mucosa is present in a Meckel's diverticulum, peptic ulceration can occur in the diverticulum itself or in the adjacent ileum.

D. & E. FALSE Peptic ulcers are not .found in the colon or rectum.

Features of gastrin secreting tumours of the pancreas (Zollinger-Ellison syndrome) include:-

A. adenomas in other endocrine glands
B. diarrhoea
C. glycosuria
D. intractable peptic ulceration
E. origin from beta-cells of pancreatic islets.

Infarction of the small intestine can be produced by:-

A. a dissecting aneurysm of the aorta
B. embolism from the left atrium
C. occlusion of the superior mesenteric artery
D. systemic hypotension
E. the contraceptive pill.

Answers overleaf

Syst. 3 Answers

A. TRUE   About 20 per cent of patients with gastrinomas have adenomas in other endocrine glands as well—the pluriglandular syndrome of multiple endocrine adenomas. The endocrine tissues affected are, in order of frequency, pancreatic islets, parathyroids, pituitary, adrenals and thyroid. This syndrome of multiple adenomas is probably genetically determined.

B. TRUE   Diarrhoea occurs in about one third of patients. It is due to the large volume of acid gastric juice entering the small intestine and may be associated with potassium depletion and steatorrhoea.

C. FALSE   The rare pancreatic alpha-cell tumour producing glucagon can produce diabetes, but this is not a feature of hypergastrinaemia.

D. TRUE   The main feature of these tumours is the great over production of gastric secretion and the development of multiple recurrent peptic ulcers.

E. The beta-cells produce insulin.

Syst. 4 Answers

A. TRUE   Extension of a dissecting aneurysm of the aorta to reach and block off the origin of the superior mesenteric artery is an uncommon cause.

B. TRUE   Embolism secondary to heart disease is a common cause. Emboli arise from the left atrium in association with atrial fibrillation and from the left ventricle in association with myocardial infarcts.

C. TRUE   This artery normally supplies almost the whole of the small intestine, apart from the first part of the duodenum.

D. TRUE   The low cardiac output of shock is a common cause of reduced intestinal blood flow, though infarction is rare.

E. TRUE   An uncommon cause. The contraceptive pill increases the incidence of venous thrombosis. Any cause of obstruction of the intestinal venous drainage can cause infarction.

Features of regional enteritis (Crohn's disease) include:-

A. fistula formation
B. multiple discontinuous lesions (skip lesions)
C. necrosis of muscle
D. stricture formation
E. tuberculoid granulomas.

Causes of chronic pulmonary hypertension include:-

A. interatrial septal defects
B. interventricular septal defects
C. mitral stenosis
D. multiple pulmonary emboli
E. cirrhosis of the liver.

Answers overleaf

Syst. 5 Answers

A. TRUE A fairly common complication of Crohn's disease. Fistulae are of several types: between adjacent loops of bowel; between a loop of bowel and the skin of the abdominal wall; anal fistulae, not continuous with a portion of affected intestine; and rarely, between an affected loop of intestine and adjacent bladder or vagina.

B. TRUE Segments of diseased intestine with normal intervening areas are quite common.

C. FALSE Muscle necrosis does not occur—in contrast to its frequent occurrence in ischaemic lesions.

D. TRUE Fibrous strictures are quite common.

E. TRUE Non-caseating tuberculoid granulomas are a characteristic histological feature, though they are only found in about 50-60 per cent of cases.

Syst. 6 Answers

A. & B. TRUE An increased pulmonary blood flow leads to hyperkinetic pulmonary hypertension. It is due to shunting of blood from the left side of the heart or aorta to the pulmonary circulation. It can result from any congenital cardio-vascular anomaly with a septal defect or aorto-pulmonary shunt, either alone or in conjunction with other cardiac lesions. It has been observed following some surgical shunt operations for Fallot's tetralogy.

C. TRUE Mitral stenosis is an important cause of chronic passive pulmonary hypertension leading to brown induration of the lungs.

D. TRUE Mechanical obstruction of pulmonary arteries can cause pulmonary hypertension. The obstruction may be due to emboli—recurrent thrombotic emboli or rarely tumour emboli—or to external compression as in the pneumoconioses.

E. FALSE This produces *portal*, not *pulmonary*, hypertension.

Systemic hypertension is an important sequel of:-

A. chronic glomerulonephritis
B. chronic pyelonephritis
C. coarctation of the aorta
D. syphilitic aortitis
E. rheumatic heart disease.

Severe myocardial infarction is associated with:-

A. fever
B. leucocytosis
C. raised erythrocyte sedimentation rate
D. raised plasma transaminase levels
E. thrombocytopenia.

Answers overleaf

Syst. 7 Answers

A. & B. TRUE Many forms of destructive renal disease, especially if associated with renal ischaemia, lead to hypertension. Sometimes chronic pyelonephritis affects only one kidney and its removal may cure or diminish the hypertension.

C. TRUE Arterial hypertension is found in the head, neck, arms and upper thorax.

D. FALSE The important features are the development of aortic incompetence and aortic aneurysms.

E. FALSE

Syst. 8 Answers

A. TRUE A moderate transitory fever of several days' duration is common.

B. TRUE A neutrophil leucocytosis is common, and the height to which the count rises is a rough measure of the severity of the infarct.

C. TRUE

D. TRUE After myocardial infarction the activities of several enzymes in plasma increase. The aspartate transaminase (AST) shows a significant increase in 6 to 12 hours, reaches a peak at about two days and remains raised for up to a week. AST levels also increase when liver cell necrosis occurs.

E. FALSE There may even be a rise in the platelet count.

Aneurysms of the aorta can occur as a sequel of:-

A. atheroma
B. diabetic microangiopathy
C. idiopathic cystic medial necrosis
D. syphilitic aortitis
E. trauma.

Acute osteomyelitis of long bones is characteristically associated with:-

A. *Escherichia coli* infection
B. involvement of the metaphysis of the bone
C. occurrence in childhood
D. subsequent development of amyloid disease
E. subsequent development of osteosarcoma.

Answers overleaf

Syst. 9 Answers

A. TRUE   The commonest cause of aortic aneurysms. Atheromatous aneurysms chiefly affect the distal aorta.

B. FALSE   This lesion of small vessels produces capillary aneurysms in the retina and kidney.

C. TRUE   This is the basic lesion of dissecting aneurysms and of Marfan's syndrome.

D. TRUE   This is a major cause of aneurysms of the ascending aorta and aortic arch.

E. TRUE   Road traffic accidents, especially crushing from the steering wheel, may damage the aorta leading to rupture or less commonly aneurysm formation.

Syst. 10 Answers

A. FALSE   The usual infecting organism is *Staph. aureus*.

B. TRUE   This is the typical site for the infection.

C. TRUE   The majority of cases occur in childhood.

D. TRUE   Amyloidosis is a recognised complication of long-standing chronic osteomyelitis.

E. FALSE   Rarely, however, a squamous cell carcinoma may develop in the skin margin of a chronic osteomyelitic sinus.

Factors of importance in producing osteoporosis are:-

A. immobilisation
B. glucocorticosteroid therapy
C. oestrogen therapy
D. old age
E. scurvy.

Lymph node enlargement is a feature of:-

A. sarcoidosis
B. primary syphilis
C. secondary syphilis
D. tertiary syphilis
E. *Yersinia enterocolitica* (*Pasteurella pseudotuberculosis*) infection.

Answers overleaf

Syst. 11 Answers

A. TRUE Immobilisation or prolonged recumbency leads to a steady loss of bone calcium.

B. TRUE Prolonged administration of these drugs produces all the features of Cushing's syndrome including osteoporosis. Pathological fractures may then ensue.

C. FALSE There is some evidence to suggest that osteoporosis may result from oestrogen deficiency as in post-menopausal osteoporosis.

D. TRUE Osteoporosis occurs in the aged of both sexes.

E. TRUE Vitamin C is essential for the formation of collagen and of osteoid tissue.

Syst. 12 Answers

A. TRUE Lymph nodes are commonly affected.

B. TRUE The regional nodes draining the primary chancre become enlarged and hard.

C. TRUE There is usually a systemic upset with skin rashes and a moderate generalised enlargement of lymph nodes.

D. FALSE The nodes are rarely directly affected at this stage.

E. TRUE This organism produces acute mesenteric lymphadenitis.